Occupational Therapy Approaches for Secondary Special Needs

Practical Classroom Strategies

Occupational Therapy Approaches for Secondary Special Needs

Practical Classroom Strategies

Jill Jenkinson
Senior Occupational Therapist, Children's Centre,
Dorset County Hospital, Dorchester

Tessa Hyde
Senior Occupational Therapist, Children's Centre,
Royal United Hospital, Bath

and

Saffia Ahmad
Senior Occupational Therapist, Children's Centre,
Royal United Hospital, Bath

Consulting Editor in Occupational Therapy
Clephane Hume

WHURR PUBLISHERS
London & Philadelphia

© 2002 Whurr Publishers

Whurr Publishers Ltd
19b Compton Terrace, London N1 2UN, England and
325 Chestnut Street, Philadelphia PA 19106, USA

Reprinted 2003

British Library Cataloguing in Publication Data

A catalogue record for this book is available from the
British Library.

ISBN 1 86156 330 2

Printed and bound in the UK by Hobbs the Printers,
Southampton, UK.

Contents

Contents

Foreword

Teachers in the 21st century are expected to be able to perform miracles. First, they are required to be up-to-date in their major subjects, even though, not only in fields like science and technology, millions of new articles and books on a host of relevant topics are being published around the world. Secondly, they are supposed to be abreast of all new initiatives on policy and practice that flow incessantly from governments, agencies of one kind or another, websites and their own professional bodies. On top of all this they have to try to differentiate in the way they teach their classes, treating pupils as individuals, and giving consideration to each child's ability, disposition and prior experience.

Special educational needs is an area of expertise that almost every teacher has had to pick up on the job. Few have been given the opportunity to detach themselves from their classroom for sustained professional development. Teachers become buskers, having to improvise and invent, often in mid-lesson, because no one is willing to release them for the time it would take to become an expert. In these circumstances it would be surprising if every decision and every practice were always entirely appropriate. Mistakes are bound to be made and some could turn out to be crucial.

That is why this book is so valuable. Few, if any, classroom teachers could possibly have acquired the combined professional expertise of the three authors on matters such as medical conditions from which children may suffer, the way these might affect their performance and learning in different subjects and settings, the many ways in which intervention may help, and the vast number of tried and tested practical ideas that are available. All these issues are well covered in the text.

What is particularly helpful is the clear layout, which allows non-experts to pick a way through and see what might be possible in their own classrooms. It is light years ahead of the ill-founded tips and palliatives that are sometimes offered to teachers. That clarity, plus a readable text, which neither patronises nor assumes too much expert knowledge, makes this a most valuable book of resources which should benefit anyone looking to improve classroom practice for all children, especially for those who are up against it.

Professor EC Wragg
University of Exeter

Acknowledgements

We would like to thank our families, friends and colleagues for their constant support and endless encouragement over several years. Working in multi-disciplinary teams at the Children's Centres in Dorchester and Bath, we have been able to draw upon the expertise of numerous professionals.

This book evolved from the Wessex National Association of Paediatric Occupational Therapists (NAPOT) Mainstream Working Party: original members of that group were also instrumental in getting this project off the ground. We have appreciated the on going interest of Janet Davis, Karen Dyson and Sue Lever, and the regular contributions from Lucy Kingdon which encouraged us to continue when we were overwelmed by the enormity of the task.

We are most grateful to many of our friends and colleagues for their help and support: to Mandy Harris for her time, unstinting effort and IT skills when our computer competency was lacking, and to Jane Bryant and Kathy Mitchell for their constructive comments following proof reading. Specialist input was received in a number of areas and we are indebted to Lisa Johnson for help with the ICT section; to Alison Reevey for advice on Autistic Spectrum Disorder and for allowing us to use the work schedule she has developed; Keith Holland for his advice and contribution on vision; to Jane Taylor for advice on handwriting; and to Moira Byrne for her illustrations. Alison Clements spent many hours in her role as SENCO field-testing sections of the book within a secondary school setting: her constructive feedback was fundamental to its final format.

From the outset we would not have been able to initiate this project without financial support from the Wessex NAPOT Regional Group. We would also like to thank the NAPOT National Executive Committee for funding the indexing of this book, and Felicity McElderry who, in her role as Professional Advisor to NAPOT, and also as a respected and valued colleague, has generously shared her expertise, given us encouragement and helped to promote this project.

Finally we would like to acknowledge the support of our employers, the West Dorset General Hospitals NHS Trust and the Royal United Hospital NHS Trust, and also our students who have taught us so much.

The authors acknowledge that the management approach and practical solution mentioned in the text are not exhaustive and they cannot take responsibility for their use. They have also used most but not all equipment listed and cannot accept any responsibility for its use.

Introduction

Accessing the curriculum at secondary level

The awareness of special educational needs has developed rapidly during recent years, partly driven by successive legislation. This has formalized the assessment and monitoring of children and young people particularly in mainstream schools. Procedures leading to clearer identification of needs have been specified in Codes of Practice and other guidance, while the right to equal opportunities is now enshrined in the Special Educational Needs and Disability Act, 2001. There will be an increasing move to mainstream inclusion for young people with a range of needs.

How to meet those needs adequately in the context of limited resources is a major challenge to both teachers and therapists. Issues include the requirement to support not only students with physical disabilities but also those with 'low incidence' needs, which are often complex and can have a widespread impact on learning. Significant curriculum differentiation may be required. The introduction of the National Curriculum has created the potential for more standardized assessment and target-setting but has produced its own demands – not least how to make the key stages as accessible as possible, both physically and cognitively, to students with widely differing learning profiles. Concerns may relate to helping students with severe physical disabilities move around safely, and it is necessary to ensure that risk assessments are thorough. The perceived pressures of the National Curriculum may restrict opportunities for life skills and independence training, both of which are so important to young people moving out into wider communities.

Role of the paediatric occupational therapist

Meeting the needs of these students has become a team effort, with a number of professionals contributing skills to help students reach their full potential. The particular role of the paediatric occupational therapist is to identify how psychological or learning difficulties affect functional skills and to help improve these skills or develop compensatory approaches. Occupational therapy brings an understanding of the implications that certain medical conditions have for classroom learning and the remediation and management strategies required. They need to be closely interwoven with existing teaching approaches to help the student achieve his or her educational potential.

Occupational therapists assess a student's functional abilities in many areas including:

- **Gross motor skills** – postural control, mobility, balance, co-ordination

- **Fine motor skills** – eye–hand co-ordination, writing, using scissors, computer keyboard

- **Sensory and perceptual skills** – body and spatial awareness, eg. visual discrimination

- **Cognitive skills** – attention and concentration, organization and sequencing, memory

- **Personal care skills** – eating/drinking, dressing, use of toilet

- **Social/emotional skills** – self-esteem, relating to others, interpreting social cues

It is important to recognize that deficits in these areas can have a significant impact on the student's learning across the school curriculum – as much on perceptual and cognitive skills for literacy and maths as on coping with the physical environment or developing social interaction skills.

Although the number of paediatric occupational therapists is gradually increasing, there are still very few and referral rates continue to rise. As well as providing direct treatment, occupational therapists have always worked in a consultative role and are keen to enhance opportunities for students by sharing knowledge with colleagues, especially teaching staff.

The greater understanding of what paediatric occupational therapy can offer has to a large extent mirrored this development. Occupational therapists recognize the contribution that they can make to enable students to learn successfully in the school setting and teachers increasingly request this support. Working within a variety of settings, occupational therapists often place a high emphasis on early intervention. Work places include community paediatric services, child development centres, social services, schools, child and adolescent mental health teams, special schools, or private practice. Since resources are limited, by the time students start in secondary schools, they may have little or no direct access to occupational therapy.

Local services

The range of services available in each locality will vary depending on funding, specialist skills and staffing establishments. Some Local Education Authorities (LEAs), or Education Library Boards in Northern Ireland, have advisory teams for physical disabilities, sensory impairment, behavioural support and information communication technology whilst other areas have very few specialist personnel. Health service provision also varies and may include occupational therapists, physiotherapists, speech and language therapists, doctors and clinical psychologists, whilst other areas may have only a skeleton team. Some professionals work individually whilst others are part of multidisciplinary and/or inter-agency teams. The current trend towards 'joined-up working' is leading to increased collaboration between health, social services and local education authorities with the aim of producing a seamless service for young people and their families.

Expectations for students

The expectations for students transferring from primary to secondary school can be great. They generally leave a small, close-knit school to become a member of a much larger community. As students progress through the school system the content of the curriculum increases in complexity at a time when they are expected to have already developed the necessary underlying skills. Students are required to work independently in a more demanding physical and social environment, which can increase pressure if earlier skills are not well consolidated.

There can be an intense psychological effect on students who continue to experience difficulties whilst watching their peer group moving ahead with seeming ease. This may be an extremely vulnerable time for students who are susceptible to additional pressures such as teasing and bullying. Low self-esteem can undermine the efforts made in compensating for their difficulties. Students may give up if specialist help and support are not available.

As a result of inclusion policies, students who might previously have been in special schools with access to life skills programmes, are now being included in mainstream schools where it can be harder to find the time to focus on these areas.

Development of this book

Close liaison with Special Educational Needs Co-ordinators (SENCOs), or Learning Support Services in Scotland, has highlighted the need for clarification of links between students' functional abilities, their behaviour in the classroom and their educational performance. This awareness resulted in collaborative work between occupational therapists throughout the Wessex region specializing in developmental paediatrics at secondary level in order to collate:

● background information on the most commonly seen medical conditions in the classroom;
● the link between skill deficits highlighted through occupational therapy assessment and the functional performance throughout the curriculum;

- management approaches/practical strategies to address these functional difficulties;
- sources of further information.

A small working party of members from the Wessex Branch of the National Association of Paediatric Occupational Therapists (NAPOT) undertook the development of this information to provide a more widely accessible resource, that forms the basis of this book.

The book is designed to be used as a resource manual, rather than a text book and there is considerable repetition to enable quick and easy access to information and to allow each section to stand alone. The information in this book can also be used to help identify students' needs when gathering evidence for referral to outside agencies.

Working in partnership

Referral routes vary from area to area but can generally be clarified by contacting the Local Education Authority or Occupational Therapy Department at the local hospital, which will be able to give further details of paediatric services including any local training courses.

Therapists recognize the increasing demands placed on teachers and support staff to deliver the curriculum and achieve results. In addition, teachers are often limited by inadequate resources, difficulty accessing external specialists, time constraints and sometimes lack of understanding on the part of some colleagues or parents. The authors acknowledge the limitation of what any one professional can achieve and therefore emphasize the importance of partnership and collaborative working in the best interest of the student. It is essential to recognize that the United Kingdom is a multi-cultural society and that each student has specific needs and values which must be taken into consideration.

Links between school and home are vitally important and an explanation of the student's needs and helpful approaches should be shared with parents and carers. The introduction of the Parent Partnership scheme will further assist these links. Evaluating the effectiveness of support and intervention with students themselves, as well as their families and those working with them, is central to planning positive ways forward. The need to build partnerships between young people, occupational therapists, teachers and careers advisory services is also critical to supporting young people as they move on to further education and employment.

How to use this book

This book is designed as a reference manual to be 'dipped into' rather than read from 'cover to cover'. It will give a quick and easy way of identifying students' problems and provide alternative strategies for enhancing their classroom performance.

Paediatric occupational therapists observe and assess foundation skills, so this is the central theme in the book and each section relates back to these skills (see Figure I.1). It can be used in several ways:

- For a student with a RECOGNIZED MEDICAL CONDITION who is entering school, refer to Chapter 2: **MEDICAL CONDITIONS** and look up the specific condition to see how this will affect their performance.

- For a student having DIFFICULTIES ACCESSING A PARTICULAR SUBJECT, refer to Chapter 3: **CURRICULUM SUBJECTS** to see how their performance will be affected.

- The **FOUNDATION SKILLS** (Chapter 1) define the necessary skills, explain why students need to acquire them, outline the IMPLICATIONS FOR SKILL deficits and gives remediation ideas for intervention.

- The **OCCUPATIONAL THERAPY SHEETS**, cross-referenced in the text, give further PRACTICAL IDEAS. They are designed to augment any existing occupational therapy programme.

- The **APPENDICES** contains CHECKLISTS, WORK SCHEDULE and STUDENT PROFILE SHEETS to target specific deficit skill areas and implement strategies.

- The **EQUIPMENT RESOURCES** sheets are cross-referenced in the text and give details of EQUIPMENT AND SUPPLIERS.

- The **GLOSSARY** explains MEDICAL TERMS used in this book.

- For a student displaying SPECIFIC BEHAVIOURS CAUSING CONCERN, refer to the **GRID SHEET** (see overleaf) to look up possible deficit foundation skills.

Foundation skills grid sheet

This grid has been developed as a quick reference for teachers easily to identify the deficits in foundation skill areas potentially causing the students' behaviour seen in the classroom.

Teacher observations and concerns

Cannot sit still/fidgets

Slouches/falls off chair/stool

Bumps into people/things/trips and falls

Poor stamina/low energy levels

Poor handwriting/pencil skills

Difficulty manipulating instruments/tools

Poor presentation of work

Problems copying from board/book

Poor reading fluency

Difficulty finding information from graphs/tables

Poor spelling

Problems taking notes

Cannot make models

Difficulty with recall or concepts

Cannot find way round school

Problems with whole day planning

Forgets homework

Often late

Dishevelled appearance

Disorganized and never ready

Distractable and does not attend

Cannot follow verbal instructions

Off task

Socially isolated

Does not partake in group discussions

Gross motor	Motor planning	Mobility	Postural stability & balance	Body awareness	Sensory processing	Fine motor	Visual motor integration	Occular motor	Hand function	Bilateral integration	Visual perception	Spatial relationships	Form constancy	Closure	Figure ground	Visual/sequential memory	Auditory processing	Attention and listening	Understanding language	Expressive language	Auditory memory	Organization	Social interaction
		●	●	●			●							●			●						
		●	●	●													●						
●	●	●	●	●			●				●						●					●	●
	●	●						●									●						
●		●		●			●	●	●	●	●	●	●	●	●				●	●		●	
●		●		●			●	●	●	●	●							●				●	
●		●		●			●	●	●	●	●	●	●		●			●	●			●	●
		●					●	●			●	●	●	●	●		●					●	
							●	●			●	●	●		●	●		●		●			
●							●	●			●				●	●		●		●		●	
																●		●		●			
		●		●			●	●	●							●		●	●	●	●	●	
●		●					●	●	●	●	●	●	●	●	●		●	●		●		●	
							●	●					●		●		●	●		●			
●							●				●		●	●	●					●		●	
●																	●			●		●	
●															●			●		●		●	
●	●											●					●					●	
●				●				●	●		●				●		●					●	●
●	●						●				●	●			●		●	●				●	
			●	●			●				●	●	●	●	●		●	●	●			●	●
																	●	●		●			●
●		●		●			●								●		●	●		●		●	●
			●	●			●											●	●				●
●																		●	●	●	●	●	●

Figure I.1

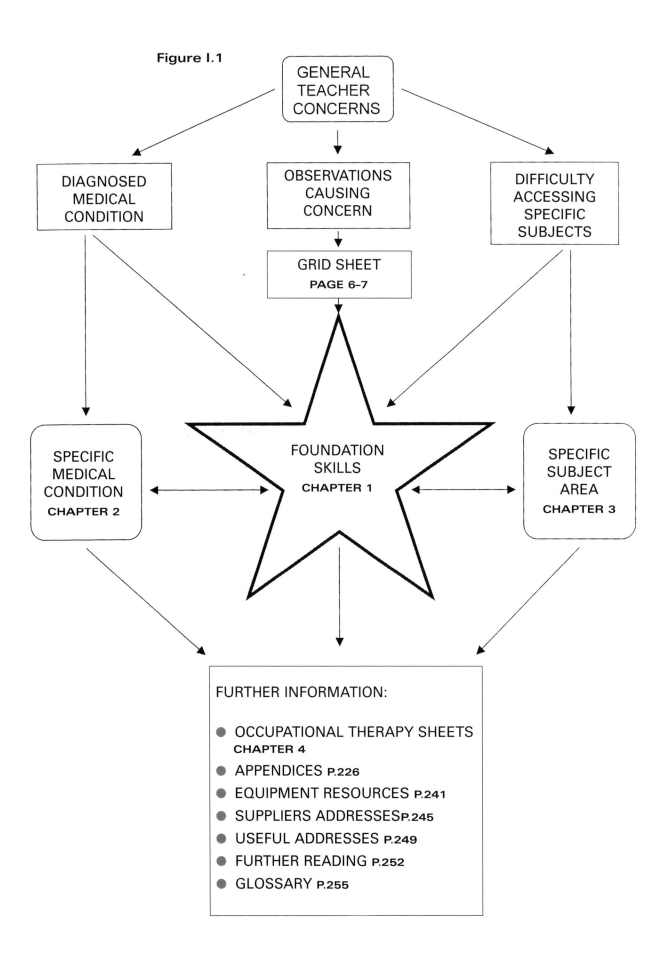

GENERAL TEACHER CONCERNS

DIAGNOSED MEDICAL CONDITION

OBSERVATIONS CAUSING CONCERN

DIFFICULTY ACCESSING SPECIFIC SUBJECTS

GRID SHEET
PAGE 6–7

SPECIFIC MEDICAL CONDITION
CHAPTER 2

FOUNDATION SKILLS
CHAPTER 1

SPECIFIC SUBJECT AREA
CHAPTER 3

FURTHER INFORMATION:

● OCCUPATIONAL THERAPY SHEETS
  CHAPTER 4
● APPENDICES P.226
● EQUIPMENT RESOURCES P.241
● SUPPLIERS ADDRESSES P.245
● USEFUL ADDRESSES P.249
● FURTHER READING P.252
● GLOSSARY P.255

Chapter 1

Foundation skills

Introduction

The particular role of the paediatric occupational therapist is to identify how physical, psychological or learning difficulties affect a child's functional skills, and to help remediate these effects or develop compensatory approaches.

Foundation skills are the developmental building blocks for learning, therefore deficits in any area will have a considerable impact on classroom performance. It is expected that by the time a student enters secondary school the basic foundation skills are well in place ready for the next stage of learning. All early experiences contribute towards learning, but some children are unable to consolidate skills at an appropriate age and therefore enter secondary school with deficits in certain areas. Since all skills are interrelated, the delay in acquiring one basic skill will have a knock-on effect for many others. For example, to develop mature pencil grasp, the student requires good gross motor co-ordination, adequate processing of sensory information (visual, tactile, auditory, proprioceptive and kinaesthetic), efficient motor planning and fine manual dexterity.

Since students use visual, motor and auditory processing skills daily and visual perceptual skills peak at puberty, every opportunity should be sought to develop innovative and interesting ways of improving a student's skills during their first three years at secondary school. It is essential to allocate regular time for Learning Support Staff to work on enhancing foundation skill development. The increasing demands of the curriculum leave little time for specific skill practice, and when working towards examinations coping strategies become more important than remediation.

In the further resources chapter activities have been suggested which will help develop these skills. The supplier's name is given first and a variety of materials are listed in their catalogues. Only a few ideas have been highlighted and other suitable equipment may already be available within the school.

F1

Gross motor co-ordination

What is it?

Gross motor co-ordination is the ability to perform large movements with fluency, accuracy and precision. In order to achieve efficient gross motor co-ordination the student must have developed and integrated the following component skills: mobility, balance, co-ordination, body awareness, postural stability, bilateral integration, sensory processing and motor planning.

Why is it important?

It provides the postural control for the acquisition of mature gross and fine motor skills, which enable refinement of integration of these skills.

What are the implications?

Students with gross motor problems may have difficulties with:

- organizing body movements;
- practical lessons;
- performance in PE;

- maintaining a functional working position;
- sitting on a high stool without a back support;
- undertaking tasks requiring stamina/standing tolerance;

- moving around the classroom/laboratory;
- carrying equipment;
- reduced stamina for extended periods of writing;
- producing an acceptable quantity of written work.

Remediation activities for gross motor skills

- Refer to Occupational Therapy sheets:

  Upper body strengthening, see **OT6**;

  Functional sitting position, see **OT1**;

  Functional working position in standing, see **OT1**.

- Refer to appendices:
  Information communication technology in the classroom, see **A3**.

Further resources for remediation

Elphinston J, Pook P (1998) The Core Workout – A Definitive Guide to Swiss Ball Training for Athletes, Coaches and Fitness Professionals. Fleet: Core Workout, Rugby Science.

Nash-Wortham M, Hunt J (1997) Take Time, Movements and Exercises for Parents, Teachers and Therapists of Children with Difficulties in Speaking, Reading, Writing and Spelling, 4th edn. Stourbridge: The Robinswood Press.

Russell JP (1988) Graded Activities for Children with Motor Difficulties. Cambridge: University Press.

Fine motor dexterity

What is it?

Fine motor dexterity is the ability to perform small, precise hand movements with fluency and accuracy. It is based on efficient development of a variety of foundation skills, e.g. proprioception, tactile processing, proximal stability and muscle strength.

Why is it important?

It facilitates the development of mature functional hand grasps.

What are the implications?

Students with fine manual dexterity problems may have difficulties with:

- handwriting – neatness, fluency and speed;
- graphics and drawing;
- presentation – labelling diagrams and maps;

- handling and operating equipment and materials;
- using tools in design technology;
- manipulating instruments - ruler, scissors, compass, tweezers, computer mouse;
- performing practical tasks – model making;

- dressing skills, e.g. small shirt buttons, tying a tie, shoe laces;
- confidence – acutely aware of their lack of ability compared to their peer group;
- frustration – give up easily.

Remediation activities for fine motor dexterity

- Refer to Occupational Therapy sheets:

    Posture/handwriting/pencil and paper tasks, see **OT1**;

    Rules for writing tasks, see **OT3**;

    Relaxation techniques for the writing hand, see **OT4**;

    Advice for left-handed students, see **OT2**;

    Hand strengthening, see **OT5**;

    Upper body strengthening, see **OT6**.

Further resources for remediation

Galt, e.g. Constucto straws
Happy Puzzle Company, e.g. Wikki Stix, Speedy Fingers, Magna Force
Levine KJ (1991) Fine Motor Dysfunction, Therapeutic Strategies in the Classroom. Tucson, AZ: Therapy Skill Builders
Novelty toys, e.g. stress balls, hole punches, Chinese balls
Physio Med, Nottingham Rehab, e.g. Therapeutic putty
Promedics (North Coast Medical), e.g. Yes-U-Can, Kids-Can-Too

---

F3 Organizational skills

What are they?

Essential components of organization are motor planning, body awareness, timing and memory. Every new task involves motor planning when the brain has to conceive of, organize and carry out a sequence of unfamiliar actions.

Why are they important?

Organizational skills influence the student's ability to organize him- or her-self in different daily and learning activities.

What are the implications?

Students with organizational problems may have difficulties with:

- organization of self and/or belongings;
- preparing for the school day;
- having correct equipment available;
- organizing work area/desk;

- presentation and layout of work;
- performing practical tasks;
- using ICT;

- PE/outdoor activities and field trips;
- tidy appearance;
- poor time keeping/forgetfulness – often in the wrong place at the wrong time;
- poor self-esteem and vulnerability to teasing.

Remediation activities for organizational skills

- Refer to Occupational Therapy sheet 'Self-organization', see **OT7**.
- Refer to Appendix work schedule, see **A5**.
- Give additional instructions and monitor the use of school diary.
- Use buddy scheme to assist confidence.
- Use school locker and checklist.
- Use computer/laptop for neat presentation of project work.

Further resources for remediation

Davis L (1996) Study Strategies Made Easy, A Practical Plan for School Success. Florida: Speciality Press.
Mind mapping e.g.: Buzant (1989) Use Your Head. London: BBC Publications.
Lewis M, Wray D (1998) Writing across the Curriculum: Frames to Support Learning. Reading: University of Reading, Reading and Language Information Centre.
The Right Brain series. Belford: Ann Arbor Publishers. (Out of print.)
Wray D, Lewis M (1997) Extending Literacy. London: Routledge.

Occupational Therapy Approaches for Secondary Special Needs © Whurr Publishers Ltd 2002

A brief introduction to perception: vision, touch, hearing, smell and taste F4

Each of our senses opens a different aspect of the world to us. The skills that we develop through the efficient use of our senses are called perceptual skills. These become the building blocks for healthy development, the foundation for our cognitive and reasoning skills.

Visual perception

Visual perceptual skills develop from the first weeks of life through to adolescence, by which time the full range of basic skills should be consolidated. The normal developmental growth patterns of early childhood establish the essential concepts through experiences of vertical and horizontal axes, depth, speed and directional judgements, both at rest and in motion. On this foundation, skills in both two-dimensional (2D) and three-dimensional (3D) perception develop. 2D skills can be formally assessed in categories such as: visual discrimination, visual memory, visual sequential memory, visual spatial relationships, visual figure ground, visual form constancy and visual closure. 3D perception can also be formally assessed by tasks such as block construction, but difficulties may also be evident in functional skills such as road safety, moving smoothly through a busy environment, or packing assorted items into a school bag. Further information on visual perceptual skills is given in the following pages of this chapter. Occupational therapists, in conjunction with educational psychologists, are able to assess these skills.

Tactile perception

It is easy to underestimate the importance of our *tactile* system and the problems that inadequate or distorted perceptions can cause. External stimuli such as heat or cold, light or heavy pressure, texture and pain have to be sorted and assimilated. On this foundation, discrimination of shape, size, weight and density develop. As the child learns to seek information by touch, inhibition of unwanted sensory stimulation must also take place if he or she is not to be confused and distracted by sensory overload. For example tactile figure ground awareness of clothing during dressing allows them to put on their clothing comfortably, but sensory inhibition then permits them to move on to other activities undistracted by sensory arousal from their clothes.

Proprioception is an additional and inter-linked area of tactile perception, which relates to the awareness of the body in space. Information is gained from muscles, tendons and joints, gravitational pull and balance receptors. *Vestibular* skills relate specifically to our posture and balance mechanisms. The awareness of the body in motion is our *kinaesthetic* sense and repetition of planned movements establishes motor memories. Visual-motor activity needs to be integrated into postural balance and fluency of movement.

The stability and control we have over body posture and movement, and the control we are able to exercise in adapting to our environment, have an enormous impact on our ability to learn. Occupational therapists and physiotherapists are able to assess these skills.

Auditory perception

As with other senses, a wide range of essential skills develops through efficient integration of auditory stimulation. Figure ground skills enable us to listen to a particular sound without being distracted by background noise. Short- and long-term memory are fundamental to learning. Sounds, rhythms and intonation must be discriminated, distance and direction interpreted. Correct sequencing also underpins effective communication. Speech and language therapists are able to assess auditory perceptual development, sometimes in conjunction with occupational therapists.

Management of perceptual deficits

A good assessment of perceptual development enables us to identify specific areas of difficulty so that therapy or educational programmes can be targeted more accurately.

Since visual perceptual skills peak during puberty, remediation is most effective when students initially enter secondary school and activities to help develop skills should be given at that time. However, when preparing for external examinations coping strategies should be explored with the student and these strategies should become part of the daily routine.

Teaching should be through a multisensory approach, whereby students are encouraged to verbalize what they are doing, look carefully whilst undertaking the task and try to feel their body movement. This provides auditory, visual, tactile and kinaesthetic feedback, which in turn reinforces more efficient performance.

Vision and ocular motor control[1]

What is it?

Vision is the act or power of sensing with the eyes. The visual system is a neural network that consists of two information-gathering devices (the eyes) which must co-ordinate effortlessly to obtain a single unified and clear image for transmission via the optic nerves to the visual cortex.

Why is it important?

Links between the ocular motor system and the tactile and proprioceptive systems also provide accurate spatial information to allow correct and efficient body posturing and motor control. Given that 85% of our knowledge of the world around us is obtained through vision, correct operation of the system is crucial for efficient functioning.

What are the implications?

Students with vision and ocular-motor problems may have difficulties with:

- visual stress (headaches and eye strain);
- discomfort with close work;
- fatigue, tiredness and loss of concentration;
- screwing up of the eyes, squinting and closing or covering one eye when working;

- distractibility when working;
- avoidance of close work;
- abnormal postures when reading or writing often with very short working distances;
- blurring and/or doubling of print – particularly when tired;
- keeping place and/or line when reading unless using a marker;

- copying, either from book to paper or from board to paper;
- reading comprehension or accuracy;
- handwriting – poor spacing, erratic use of lines, fatigue;
- spelling;
- co-ordination in ball games, team games or in spatial awareness.

---

1   Information taken from a study day, run by Keith Holland, Behavioural Optometrist, Cheltenham 'Visual factors and occupational therapy', 1996 and from personal correspondence.

Remediation activities for ocular motor control

- Looking up, down, left and right with the eyes only and no head movement (10 times at the start of a lesson), to stimulate simple tracking.
- Reading first and last letters on every line of a page of text or the first letter of every word, to develop saccadic eye movements needed for reading.
- Reading aloud whilst moving the material in and out and in circles, to help develop stable focus.
- Encourage pattern copying, using increasingly complex shapes to develop visual analysis skills.
- Word searches, pattern games, e.g. Battleships, Tangrams.
- Encourage visualization, e.g. daydreaming then describing the dreams with as much sensory detail as possible.
- Experiment with different coloured overlays to minimize visual stress.

Possible strategies

Visual breaks are essential and may need to be scheduled every five minutes for some students.

- Avoid peripheral distractions.
- Refer to checklist for visual signs – see Appendix, **A4**.

- Ensure good posture – see Occupational Therapy skill sheet **OT1** and **OT3**.
- Check book/paper position to find optimum working distance (i.e. equal to the distance from the elbow to the knuckle).
- Check whether angled surface is needed for comfortable working see Occupational Therapy skill sheet **OT1**.
- Sit facing the board to eliminate need to turn body.

- Ensure as much natural lighting as possible.
- Reduce time spent on close work.
- Use computers to reduce amount of handwriting required.
- Provide paper copy of information on board.
- Enlarge worksheets to ease focus demands.

- Use line trackers – refer to Equipment resources **ER**.
- Provide clear line guide drawn on overhead projector acetate.
- When interpreting data, use ruler/paper guide/'L' shaped guide.
- When scanning, reinforce working left to right, top to bottom and use margin as a reference point.

Further resources for remediation

Behavioural optometists use lenses and vision training to facilitate the development of a more efficient and complete visual process. Early detection of visual difficulties is vital, but should not rely on simple school eye tests, which are not designed to pick up these difficulties. A full optometric or behavioural optometry examination should be carried out wherever possible – consult www.babo.co.uk.

Should difficulties be found, they may be helped through the use of spectacles, vision therapy exercise programmes (usually administered by an optometrist), or by employing compensatory strategies such as the use of computers to reduce handwriting, coloured overlays to minimize visual stress or reduced time spent on close work.

Further information

British Association of Behavioural Optometrists

72 High Street
Billericay
Essex CM12 9BS
Tel: 01277 624916
email: aquila72@aol.com
www.babo.co.uk

References for further reading

Holland K (1995a) Visual Skills for Learning in Topic, Spring, No 13., pp. 1–7. NFER Nelson
Holland K (1995b) Vision for writing, Handwriting Review 9: 92-98: Handwriting Interest Group.
Wachs H, Frith H (1975) Thinking Goes to School. New York: Oxford University Press.
Willows D, Kruk R, Corcos E (1993) Visual Processed in Reading and Disabilities. London: Lawrence Erlbaum Associates.

F6   Visual motor integration

What is it?

Visual motor integration is the degree to which visual perception and finger–hand movements are well co-ordinated (Beery 1997), in order to translate visual information into a motor response.

Why is it important?

It is the foundation for the development and refinement of handwriting and graphic skills.

What are the implications?

Students with visual motor integration problems may have difficulties with:

- handwriting and recording tasks although verbal skills are good;
- copying either from book to paper or from board to paper;
- graphics and drawing tasks;
- spacing and staying on lines;
- presentation of work, e.g. labelling diagrams and maps;

- inaccurate erasing of own work;
- performing practical activities, e.g. using scissors or microscope, building models;
- manipulating instruments;
- PE, e.g. ball skills, team games, apparatus work.

Remediation activities for visual motor integration

- Refer to vision and ocular motor control skill sheet, see **F5**.
- Origami, paper folding, craft activities.
- Copying drawings and locating grid positions.
- Find the shortest route on maps/mazes.
- Tracing activities.
- Word searches.
- Directional drawings with eyes closed, e.g. follow verbal directions; 'up stop', 'to the right stop'. Draw: shapes, letters, words with eyes closed, from verbal instructions.
- Picture/word matching card games.
- Introduction of laptop in conjunction with touch typing software to improve typing skills for recording work. See Appendix **A3**.

Occupational Therapy Approaches for Secondary Special Needs © Whurr Publishers Ltd 2002

Further resources for remediation

Ann Arbor Publishers Ltd. e.g.:

Jay Lev L (1975) Eye-Hand Boosters. Novato, CA: Academic Therapy Publishers.

Jay Lev L (1988) Eye-Hand Coordination Boosters. A book of 92 Blackline masters. Novato, CA: Academic Therapy Publishers.

McCreary P (1997) The Maze Book. Novato, CA: Ann Arbor Publishers.

Perceptual Activities (2001) Novato, CA: Ann Arbor Publishers.

Relevant computer software.

Tarquin, e.g. Altair Design, Geoboards

Teodorescu I, Addy LM (1996) Write from the Start, the Teodorescu Perceptual-Motor Programme – Developing the fine motor and perceptual skills for effective handwriting. Wisbech: LDA.

References

Beery KB (1997) Developmental Test of Visual Motor Integration VMI, New Jersey, NJ: Modern Curriculum Press.

F7 Visual spatial relationships

What are they?

Visual spatial perception provides us with information about the position of two or more objects in relation to self and each another.

Why is it important?

Some students experience difficulty in appreciating and processing spatial information from their environment. Inadequate spatial perception has an impact on a student's learning; at secondary level the student's ability to interpret and use perspective is often impaired.

What are the implications?

Students with visual spatial relationship problems may experience difficulties with:

- managing stairs, kerbs;
- moving in space, e.g. team games, PE, improvization in dance/drama;
- staying within personal boundaries and understanding personal space;
- learning left/right;

- reversing letters/numbers;
- handwriting – size, shape, spacing of letters, writing on the line;
- other pencil and paper activities – copying pictures, drawing plans, labelling diagrams;
- setting out work on a page;

- linear and vertical scanning;
- understanding scale, using and interpreting drawings, maps;
- constructing a model or setting up an experiment from a diagram (2D-3D) or drawing diagram from model (3D-2D);
- understanding size, angle, depth, height, orientation.

Remediation activities for visual spatial relationships

- Refer to vision and ocular motor control skill sheet, see **F5**.
- Mazes, dot to dot, word searches.
- Copying activities: 3D-3D, 2D-3D, 2D-2D and 3D-2D.
- Drawing simple maps.
- Reading grid references on maps using vertical and linear scanning.

Occupational Therapy Approaches for Secondary Special Needs © Whurr Publishers Ltd 2002

- Using 1cm squared paper to draw lines from one point to another, gradually reducing the size of the squares.
- Use isometric/lattice grid papers.

Further resources for remediation

Ann Arbor Publishers, e.g. Right brain series
ASCO, e.g. Pyramis
The Happy Puzzle Company, e.g. Rush Hour, Happy Cubes, Block by Block, ABC Blocks
HOPE/Galt, e.g. Knex, Meccano
LDA, e.g. Let's Look, Pattern Blocks Puzzle Trays, Spatial Relationship Lotto
Relevant computer software
Tarquin, e.g. Dime Solids, Build-up, Tri-cube, Pentacubes, Tangrams
Taskmaster, e.g. Mathematics Through Paper Folding

F8 Visual form constancy

What is it?

Visual form constancy is the ability to recognize the fact that a shape remains the same despite changes in size, direction orientation and distance, e.g. an object is still the same whether it is seen from the top or side.

Visual memory, figure ground skills and visual discrimination may all contribute to establishing form constancy.

Why is it important?

It represents the ability of the individual to interpret the environment consistently and accurately regardless of changes in presentation of the information.

What are the implications?

Students with visual form constancy problems may experience difficulties with:

- categorizing and classifying objects/shapes/materials;
- sorting, especially when orientation and shape change;
- obtaining measurements and investigating properties of scale;
- generalizing concepts about a change in size, or direction;

- constructing 3D and 2D shapes from given information;
- drawing 2D shapes in different orientation;
- recognizing and using 2D representation of 3D objects;

- transferring from printed to cursive writing;
- copying from a book;
- recognizing and reading the same word/letter when presented in different handwriting styles/fonts/typefaces.

Remediation activities for visual form constancy

- Frequently demonstrate how horizontally presented material looks when presented vertically.
- Work with concrete objects – explore properties of each object and relate to 2D representations.
- Present the same word in many different styles, types, colours, fonts together with other words. Encourage student to underline the same word presented in many different forms.
- Make 3D model from 2D diagram/picture/sketch, e.g. aeroplane, castle, volcano.

- Use orientation of objects visual cue cards to identify objects seen from different angles, e.g. from above, behind, in front, underneath.

Further resources for remediation

ASCO, e.g. Pyramis, Kit Cubes
Happy Puzzle Company, e.g. Rush Hour, Brick By Brick, Block By Block

Relevant computer software
Tarquin, e.g. Mirror puzzle, Dime solids, Tricubes, Pentacubes
Taskmaster, e.g. Geostrips

F9 Visual figure ground discrimination

What is it?

Visual figure ground discrimination is the ability to identify relevant information from a background that contains irrelevant or distracting objects/images.

Why is it important?

It is the ability to screen out irrelevant visual material in order to concentrate on the important stimulus. Students with poor visual attention often experience difficulty with figure ground discrimination.

What are the implications?

Students with visual figure ground discrimination problems may experience difficulties with:

- attending to task;
- ignoring what is irrelevant;
- concentrating on relevant stimuli;

- shifting attention appropriately;
- extracting relevant information from text, diagrams, graphs, pie charts, spreadsheets, database;
- finding specific place in text, map, manuscript line, multiple choice;

- scanning adequately, resulting in poor 'skim and scan' skills;
- noticing all the relevant words in question, identifying keywords;
- keeping place when reading, completing a worksheet or copying work from book or board;

- organizing and laying out written work;
- completing all sections in written assignments;
- interpreting and labelling diagrams/drawings.

Remediation activities for visual figure ground discrimination

- Refer to vision and ocular motor control skill sheet, see **F5**.
- Circling the same word in a text.
- Word searches.
- Jigsaw puzzles.
- Activity books, e.g. 'Where's Wally?'
- 'Odd one out' puzzles.
- I-spy games.

25

Further resources for remediation

Ann Arbor Publishers, e.g. Perceptual Activities Book, Cues and Comprehension, Number
Tracking, Multiple Tracking, Sentence Tracking

HOPE e.g. Scope 2000

Relevant computer software

Tarquin, e.g. Altair Design, Polysymetrics, Escher - Illusions and perception

F10 Visual closure

What is it?

Visual closure is the ability to see 'in the mind's eye' the whole of an object when part of it is hidden. It involves manipulating and transposing visual information. Visual closure is closely interlinked with cognitive ability and conceptualization. It allows accurate judgements to be made from familiar, but partial information.

Why is it important?

It is a foundation skill for fluency and speed in reading and spelling. Efficient reading relies on visual closure because with each fixation of the eye only part of the letters of a word or phrase is actually perceived. As a student becomes more competent in reading, eye fixations become fewer and he or she must 'fill in' more material and encompass a wider area of print.

What are the implications?

Students with visual closure problems may experience difficulties with:

- identifying a visual object from an incomplete or unclear representation;
- putting parts together to form a whole;
- visualizing images;

- spelling patterns;
- blending letters into words visually;

- putting letters together to make a word although they may be able to read the individual letters;
- mathematical calculations and multiplication tables;
- visualization of processes, e.g. 'life cycles' in biology;
- identifying components for chemistry formulas/maths equations;

- whole day planning;
- categorizing time and space.

Remediation activities for visual closure

- Refer to vision and ocular motor control skill sheet, see **F5**.
- Manipulating and rotating shapes/objects when discussing their properties.
- Finishing incomplete pictures, gradually reducing given prompts.
- Drawing a picture/shape/object then rotating it through 90 degrees – drawing it upside down, highlighting lower half, etc.

Occupational Therapy Approaches for Secondary Special Needs © Whurr Publishers Ltd 2002

F10

- Transferring a design shape from one grid to another.
- Symmetry and tessellations – completing the other half of a picture/design.
- Filling in letters to complete words or fill in words to complete sentences.

Further resources for remediation

Ann Arbor Publishers, e.g. Half 'n' Half Design and Colour
ASCO, e.g. Horizons, Geovolume
Happy Puzzle Company, e.g. Go Getter puzzles, Shape by Shape
Philip and Tacey, e.g. Geonimoes

Relevant computer software
Tarquin, e.g. Tangrams, Mind's eye geometry

F11 Visual memory/sequential memory

What is it?

Visual memory/sequential memory is the ability to remember what is seen and to recall visual images of objects, shapes, symbols and movements. It is the term used to describe how memory activity processes visual information from short-term recall into long-term store.

Why is it important?

It is a foundation skill for all learning and is essential for accuracy in copying tasks.

What are the implications?

Students with visual memory/sequential memory problems may experience difficulties with:

- remembering visual sequences and letter shapes;
- orientation of letters or numbers;
- reading and number work;
- recalling information apparently learnt previously;

- organizing work;
- concentrating and attending to task;
- making notes;

- reproducing formulas and symbols;
- reproducing data from book or board;
- recalling equations and formulas;
- remembering the sequence from a practical demonstration;
- copying musical notation/shape patterns.

Remediation activities for visual memory/visual sequential memory

- Refer to vision and ocular motor control skill sheet, see **F5**.
- Drawing pictures of story/day's events/video/TV programme.
- 2D-2D copying activities.
- Drawing and copying a repeated sequence of shapes.
- Word searches/find the differences.
- Underlining letter/number combinations in given text.
- Timed exercise copying from board to paper.

Further resources for remediation

Ann Arbor Publishers, e.g. Symbol Discrimination and Sequencing, The Maze Book
    (Paul McCreary 1997), Symbol/Letter Tracking, Right Brain series
Egon Publications, e.g. Spelling Made Easy. Violet Brand
LDA, e.g. Visual Recall Flash cards, Stile, Sequential Thinking Sets

Relevant computer software
Smart Kids (UK) Ltd, e.g. Homophones, Homographs
Taskmaster, e.g. Word Hexagons, Linkaword Endings
Winslow, e.g. Dotbot Sequencing Activities; 2,3,4 Sequences Galore

F12 Auditory processing and memory

What is it?

Auditory memory is the term used to describe how memory activity processes auditory information from short-term recall into long-term store.

Why is it important?

The function of auditory memory is to hold information, whilst it is being manipulated and processed, and to store the resulting information. There are three stages of memory – encoding, storage and retrieval – which are foundation skills for learning.

What are the implications?

Students with auditory memory and processing problems may experience difficulties with:

- focusing on and identifying key points within verbal presentations;
- blocking out background noises and other sensory information sufficiently in order to concentrate on essential instructions;
- processing auditory material at speed;
- processing a variety of styles/presentations, e.g. teaching, speaking;
- following verbal instructions;
- group discussions as unable to sift, summarize and follow conversation;
- responding to directions and completing tasks;

- appearing disorganized because unable to process instructions;
- haphazardly rushing into tasks;
- carrying out verbal instructions in the wrong order;
- word finding;
- phonological awareness and literacy;
- remembering and sequencing multiple-step instructions;
- solving mental arithmetic problems and learning multiplication tables;
- learning by rote.

Remediation activities for auditory processing and memory

- Encourage use of pictorial/written cues, provide written lesson/homework plans.
- Identify key words or facts as the lesson/instruction progresses.
- Ask student to repeat teacher's instructions.

Occupational Therapy Approaches for Secondary Special Needs © Whurr Publishers Ltd 2002

- Jot down key words or telegrammatic sentences to aid recall.
- Chinese whispers.
- Word-finding activities.

Further resources for remediation

Ann Arbor Publishers, e.g. Sound Out Listening Skills Program (Geraldine M. Kimmell),
    Auditory Processes (revised, Pamela Gillet), Right Brain Series
Egon Publishers, e.g. Sound Activities
LDA, e.g. Stile Tray, Stile Spelling and Phonics
Multi -Sensory Learning catalogue, e.g. The Association Cards
Wilson J (1994) P.A.T. Phonological Awareness Training: A New Approach to Phonics.
    London: Educational Psychology Publishing.

F13 Social interaction

What is it?

Social interaction is the ability to communicate efficiently and understand cues from social situations. It involves the ability to manoeuvre a way through the world and social situations in order to have physical and emotional needs met.

Why is it important?

Social interaction is one of the foundation skills for emotional wellbeing. It is important to communicate needs in different situations both physical and emotional, in order to develop meaningful relationships.

What are the implications?

Students with social interaction problems may have difficulties with:

- interpreting and using gesture, facial expression and body language;
- understanding the communication of emotions and feelings;
- understanding the effect of their behaviour on other students;
- self-confidence, self-esteem;

- using language appropriately;
- participating in discussions, role play, debates, conversation or even communicating basic needs;
- independence and problem-solving;

- developing a sense of self and identity in peer group;
- developing sexual identity;
- understanding the rules/boundaries of friendships;
- maintaining friendships and dealing with rejection, resolving conflict;
- understanding ambiguity and sarcasm;
- participating in team games.

Remediation activities for social interaction

- Social skills groups.
- Self-esteem groups.
- Partner and small group work, including interaction and turn-taking activities.
- Social use of language programme.

Further resources for remediation

Relevant computer software, e.g. (1) Gaining Face – CD Rom available from the National Autistic Society or www.ccoder.com; (2) Emotion Trainer – available on the internet at www.emotiontrainer.co.uk

Feeling Thermometer, Circle of Friends and Emotion Scrapbook – see Attwood T (1998) Asperger's Syndrome, A Guide for Parents and Professionals. London: Jessica Kingsley.

Gray C (2000) Writing Social Stories with Carol Gray. Arlington, TX: Future Horizons.

Gray C (1994) Comic Strip Conversations. Arlington, TX: Future Horizons.

Hodgdon L (1995) Visual Strategies for Improving Communication. Troy, MI: QuirkRoberts Publishers.

Rinaldi W (1992) The Social Use of Language Programme. Windsor: NFER Nelson.

Sainsbury C (2000) Martian in the Playground, Understanding the School Child with Asperger's Syndrome. Bristol: Lucky Duck.

Chapter 2

Medical conditions

Introduction

The current trend towards total inclusion in mainstream schools has resulted in an increasing need for teachers and school staff to understand a range of medical conditions. Students already diagnosed with a medical condition may have specific needs, which will affect their classroom performance and therefore their ability to access the National Curriculum.

Occupational therapists work with a wide range of diagnoses, often being able to follow the student through both primary and secondary school placements. Occupational therapists work with teachers and support staff to integrate students into their secondary school.

The most common medical conditions seen by paediatric occupational therapists have been identified as:

- attention deficit disorder/attention deficit hyperactivity disorder (ADD/ADHD);
- autistic spectrum disorders (ASD) including Asperger's syndrome;
- cerebral palsy (CP);
- developmental co-ordination disorder (DCD), including dyspraxia;
- dystrophies and degenerative conditions (DC);
- juvenile idiopathic arthritis (JIA).

It is now acknowledged that many conditions co-exist alongside the primary diagnosis (referred to as co-morbidity); consequently sometimes a student's presenting features may be attributable to more than one condition. This can be particularly evident in students who display features of attention deficit/attention deficit hyperactivity disorder, autistic spectrum disorder and developmental co-ordination disorder.

Teachers will be aware of students who have other medical diagnoses, and details of these conditions should be available from the school doctor, school nurse and information sources such as the *Contact a Family Directory* (see Contact a Family entry in the Useful Addresses section at the end of this book).

Treatment procedures and the personnel referred to in the text will vary depending on the medical, educational and social services networks in the local area. To ensure that a consistent approach is maintained throughout the school it is advisable that any request for further advice from outside agencies is discussed with the SENCO.

Initially a member of staff might be given the introductory front sheet to learn about the medical condition of the student being supported. Later, when familiar with the student, the tables associated with each condition covered in this book will help to identify strategies that may be effective in the different situations the student encounters.

MC1 Attention deficit disorder/attention deficit hyperactivity disorder

Definition

Attention deficit disorder/attention deficit hyperactivity disorder (ADD/ADHD) may be diagnosed in children and young persons where behaviour appears impulsive, overactive and/or inattentive to an extent that is unwarranted for their developmental age and is a significant hindrance to their social and educational successes (British Psychological Society 1996). In order to be given a clinical diagnosis of ADD/ADHD the student must be formally assessed by specialist medical practitioners and meet certain diagnostic criteria. Two major diagnostic instruments are currently used by clinicians – the Diagnostic and Statistical Manual of Mental Disorders (DSM-IV) and International Classification of Diseases, 10th edition (ICD-10).

Cause

The precise cause of ADD/ADHD cannot yet be specified, however it is hypothesized to be a neurologically based condition, resulting from a difference in brain chemistry, rather than a deficit or impairment in brain function.

What are the main forms of ADD/ADHD?

Some students display predominately inattentive/sluggish behaviour whilst others show hyperactivity/impulsive behaviour. In a few instances these features may be combined. It is seldom seen as a 'pure' diagnosis since other co-existing conditions can be present, e.g. Asperger's syndrome, developmental co-ordination disorder. When a combination of developmental co-ordination disorder and attention deficit hyperactivity disorder is present a diagnosis of DAMP, i.e. deficits in attention, motor control and perception (Gillberg 1983) may be given.

The intensity of the core symptoms can differ significantly from student to student and from one situation to another. This unevenness of symptoms may affect the student's performance within the classroom depending on the subject, the teaching method used and the timing of medication, if prescribed. Behaviour at home may vary according to normal demands of family life, social interaction, roles within the family and timing of medication, if prescribed.

Occupational Therapy Approaches for Secondary Special Needs © Whurr Publishers Ltd 2002

MC1

Presenting features

Specific characteristics and behaviour may include the following:

1 Inattention

- difficulty focusing on task, leading to careless mistakes;
- inability to sustain focus on task due to variable concentration;
- unable to follow instructions accurately through to completion of task;
- school work and homework often incomplete, because does not follow through on instructions;
- disorganized approach to work;
- frequently loses equipment, book, PE kit, etc.;
- poor selective attention and easily distracted by extraneous stimuli;
- shifting from one uncompleted task to another;
- forgetful in daily activities.

2 Hyperactivity

- tendency to fidget and fiddle;
- finds sitting still difficult – constantly 'on the move';
- frequently leaves seat in classroom;
- restless in self;
- talks excessively and is demanding in group situations.

3 Impulsiveness

- tends to make decisions hastily without considering alternatives/consequences;
- has difficulty waiting their turn;
- lacks self-control;
- poor at problem-solving.

4 Social/emotional factors

- may be 'class clown' or withdrawn;
- can become antisocial;
- inability to follow social rules in group situations;
- inappropriate social behaviours;
- poor sleeping patterns affecting behaviour at school.

Treatment

No treatment has yet been proved to cure the condition of ADD/ADHD, all provide purely symptomatic relief. However, as students get older and learn to live with this condition improvement is often noticed.

Common types of intervention include:

- medication;
- behaviour management;
- social skills training;
- self-control monitoring;
- manipulation of the environment;
- sensory modulation.

Prognosis

The symptoms continue to persist, but students can learn strategies to help them modify their behaviour.

References

British Pyschological Society (1996) Attention Deficit Hyperactivity Disorder (ADHD): A Psychological Response to an Evolving Concept. Leicester: The British Psychological Society.

Gillberg C (1983) Perceptual, motor and attention deficits in Swedish primary school children: some child psychiatric aspects. Journal of Child Psychology and Psychiatry 24: 337-403.

Reed, Cathlyn, L (2001) Quick Reference to Occupational Therapy, 2nd edn. Gaithersburg, MD: Aspen Publishers

---

Further information

ADDISS: ADD Information Services
PO Box 340
Edgeware
Middlesex HA8 9HL
Tel: 020 8906 9068
Fax: 020 8959 0727
www.addiss.co.uk

The ADDISS Resource Centre
10 Station Road
Mill Hill
London NW7 2JU
Tel: 020 8906 9068
Fax: 020 8959 0727
www.addiss.co.uk

ADD/ADHD Family Support Group
Mrs Gillian Mead
1a The High Street
Dilton Marsh
Nr. Westbury
Wiltshire BA13 4DL
Tel: 01373 826045

Further reading

Alban-Metcalfe J, Alban-Metcalfe J (2001) Managing ADHD in the Inclusive Classroom – Practical Strategies for Teachers. London: Fulton.

Barkley RA (1995) Taking Charge of ADHD – The Complete, Authoritative Guide for Parents. New York: The Guilford Press.

Cooper P, Ideus K (1996) ADHD – A Practical Guide for Teaching. London: Fulton.

Dendy CZ (2000) Teaching Teens with ADD and ADHD – A Quick Reference Guide for Teachers and Parents. Bethesda, MD: Woodbine House. (Available through ADDISS.)

Green C, Chee K (1997) Understanding ADHD – A Parent's Guide to ADHD in Children. London: Vermillion.

Goldstein S, Goldstein M (1990) Managing Attention Disorders in Children: A Guide for Practitioners. New York: John Wiley and Sons.

Jones CB (1994) Attention Deficit Disorder – Strategies for School Age Children. Tucson, AZ: Communication Skill Builders/London: Psychological Corporation.

Kewley G (2001) ADHD Recognition, Reality and Resolution. London: Fulton.

Parker H (1992) The ADD Hyperactivity Handbook for School. Chesterfield: Winslow.

Reed, Cathlyn, L., (2001) Quick Reference to Occupational Therapy. 2nd edn. Gaithersburg, MD: Aspen Publishers.

Table 2.1 ADD/ADHD

Students diagnosed with attention deficit disorder/attention deficit hyperactivity disorder will present with varying degrees of need depending on the severity of their condition. The presenting features mentioned below are an extensive list and may not all be relevant.

Management should be targeted for the individual student after an analysis of the observed behaviours. It will then be important to decide whether the behaviour needs to be managed or changed. It may be necessary to seek advice from your SENCO in order to implement some of these approaches.

Possible Presenting Features	Management Approaches	Further Advice via SENCO
Behaviour		

■ Impulsive
  blurts out answers/interrupts
  starts activity before listening to full instructions
  acts without thinking
	■ Behaviour management programme
	  Heighten teachers' and peers' awareness of student's difficulty
	  Consider adult support for group situations
	  Implement calming/relaxation techniques provided by occupational therapist
		Seek support from child and adolescent mental health service, educational psychologist, behavioural support teams

■ Persistence in activities
  distractibility during study
  frequently off task
  difficulty sustaining attention
	■ Frequent positive teacher feedback and redirection
	  Set short, attainable goals
	  Have regular breaks
	  Limit distractions – only essential items in work area
	  Consider position in class
	  Behaviour management programme	

■ Not understanding and conforming to rules	■ Behaviour management/social skills programme	
■ Changeable, unpredictable behaviour	■ Ensure any medication taken as prescribed	■ Parents Discuss with doctors and parents possibility of altering timing and dosage of medication to optimize performance
■ Inappropriate response to sensory input – auditory, tactile, visual, e.g. unable to ignore irrelevant background noises	■ Heighten staff awareness that student may under- or overreact to normal sensory input, e.g. bell Eliminate distracting stimuli, e.g. background noise, pencils on desk	■ Seek advice from occupational therapist for specific guidance
■ Failure to complete work	■ Use home/school book daily to check with tutor/SENCO Clarify expectations, e.g. structured information on what student is expected to achieve	■ Work schedule – see Appendix (**A5**)

MC1 ADD/ADHD (continued)

Possible Presenting Features	Management Approaches	Further Advice via SENCO
Physical gross motor skill		**Refer to gross motor co-ordination skill sheet (F1)**

■ Impulsiveness
  inability to sustain motor control
  fluctuating quality of movement
  difficulty executing slow rhythmical movements
  poor listening to instructions before starting activity
  difficulty awaiting turn
  interfering during team games
  reduced sense of danger
  poor sequencing and organising movements
	■ Encourage/practise slow, controlled movements
	  Help/encourage student to pre-plan movements required for task
	  Implement calming techniques provided by occupational therapist
	  Heighten awareness of safety issues and undertake risk assessments as appropriate
	  Provide opportunities for individual/partner sports
	  Consider adult support to maintain awareness of safety
		■ Seek advice from occupational therapist, physiotherapist
		
		■ Refer to school health and safety policy

■ Static balance
  difficulty executing slow, precise, controlled movements
  reduced ability to sustain balance postures
	■ Ensure student is given adequate space
	  Break down activity and practise individual component parts
		■ Refer to James Russell's *Graded Motor Activities*; Elphinston Pook, *The Core Workout* (see Further reading)

■ Co-ordination of eye/hand/foot – difficulty catching/kicking ball	■ Identify specific difficulty and practise skill Heighten awareness of teacher and peers to student's difficulty	

■ Sustaining posture
  constantly on the move
  slouching
  fidgeting/fiddling
	■ Encourage student to sit rather than stand for activities if appropriate
	  Provide propping surface when standing is essential
	  'Earth' student by providing specific spot/area, e.g. on mat, in hoop
	  Allow student to 'fiddle' with an agreed object, e.g. Blu-Tack®, stress ball
	  Check seating posture (chair/table size/height)
		■ Refer to Occupational Therapy sheet (**OT6**)
		
		■ Refer to Occupational Therapy sheet (**OT1**)

MC1

Table 2.1 ADD/ADHD

Possible Presenting Features	Management Approaches	Further Advice via SENCO
Physical fine motor dexterity		**Refer to fine motor dexterity skill sheet (F2) and visual motor integration (F6)**
■ Impulsiveness/inattention/hyperactivity rushes, compromising accuracy, e.g. writing, cutting, pouring liquids lack of awareness of safety issues untidy and poor presentation of written work variable quantity of work	■ Behaviour management programme. Set attainable goals – encourage student to slow down and monitor results. Allow short breaks to refocus during tasks. Heighten awareness of safety issues and undertake risk assessment as appropriate. Clearly reward quality rather than just quantity and finishing task.	■ Refer to Occupational Therapy sheet (**OT5**) ■ Refer to school health and safety policy
Organizational		**Refer to organizational skills sheet (F3)**
■ Inability to organize self and task acting before thinking preparation for school day and subjects	■ Consider use of work schedules. Help and encourage student to pre-plan task – stop/think/plan/do. Liaise with family/carers regarding consistent strategies to help develop routines. Behaviour management programme. Provide checklist/cue cards identifying required equipment. Promote uncluttered work space.	■ Refer to Appendix (**A5**). ■ Seek support from educational/ clinical psychologist
■ Inability to organize work area	■ Use checklists to ensure only essential items are in work area.	
■ Difficulty completing homework	■ Discuss reason with student and parents. Check timing of medication, home environment. Consider homework club. Set realistic goals. Consider use of system for recording homework.	■ Refer to Occupational Therapy sheet (**OT7**)

Occupational Therapy Approaches for Secondary Special Needs © Whurr Publishers Ltd 2002

MC1 ADD/ADHD (continued)

Possible Presenting Features	Management Approaches	Further Advice via SENCO
Organizational (continued)		
■ Limited awareness of danger/no sense of danger	■ Heighten staff awareness Raise students awareness of potential danger Paired working and/or adult support Use safety checklists	■ Refer to school health and safety policy.
■ Reduced concept of time	■ Allocate time in weekly timetable for completing essential work Adult monitoring in unstructured situations Teach coping strategies, e.g. use alarm on watches, timers, timed checklist	
Communication		**Refer to auditory processing and memory skill sheet (F13)**
■ Difficulty focusing on and responding to relevant auditory information	■ Reduce extraneous background noises Give clear, concise instructions Encourage student to repeat information back Teach strategies to improve listening skills Encourage student to take notes Use of visual cues	■ Seek advice from speech and language therapist, educational psychologist
■ Speaking before thinking	■ Teach student to stop and think before speaking Encourage student to self-check to ensure keeping on target Behaviour management programme	■ Refer to social interaction skill sheet (**F13**)
■ Fast/jumbled thoughts when speaking/writing	■ Teach mind-mapping techniques Teach self-checking skills Make notes of key points to maintain focus	■ Refer to Further Reading Seek advice from speech and language therapist, educational psychologist.

Table 2.1 ADD/ADHD

Possible Presenting Features	Management Approaches	Further Advice via SENCO
Perception		**Refer to a brief introduction to perception (F4) vision and ocular motor control skill sheet (F5)**
■ Visual perception – interpreting visual information: figure ground discrimination, e.g. finding place on board/page	■ Refer to visual figure ground discrimination skill sheet (F9)	
spatial awareness, e.g. directionality visual closure, e.g. visualization of processes, such as lifecycles in biology	Refer to visual spatial relationships skill sheet (F7) Refer to visual closure skill sheet (F10)	
■ Vision and ocular motor control – keeping focus on teacher/board copying from board following text in book/paper	■ Sit centrally in class, facing front Give individual paper copy of instructions/work written on board Use reading guide or ruler below line of print/figures in columns	■ Seek advice from occupational therapist, behavioural optometrist ■ Refer to checklist for visual signs, see Appendix (A4)
making directional changes quickly	Expect less fluency in PE activities which require continual turning/visual checking (team games)	
fuzzy/blurred print	Consider use of individual coloured overlay	
Self-care		
■ Dressing inattention and rushing poor organization	■ Behaviour management programme	
■ Road safety implications	■ Implement recommended impulsive control strategies Provide adult support	■ Seek advice from occupational therapist, child and adolescent mental health service
■ Mealtimes rushes and inattentive with all aspects of task restless standing in lunch queue messy mouth/hands/clothing after meals	■ Behaviour management programme Stand at front/back of queue Heighten staff awareness of implications, e.g. food on jumper/table Encourage student to routinely check clean hand/face and clothing after meal	

Occupational Therapy Approaches for Secondary Special Needs © Whurr Publishers Ltd 2002

MC1 ADD/ADHD (continued)

Possible Presenting Features	Management Approaches	Further Advice via SENCO
Social, emotional and psychological		**Refer to social interaction skill sheet (F13)**
■ Forming and maintaining peer relationships	■ Explanation to peer group of ADD/ADHD if student gives consent Social skills training programme Facilitate 'circle of friends' scheme	
■ Coping with unstructured situations	■ Establish clear boundaries Ensure environment and task are as structured as possible Consider adult/buddy support	
■ Working with others, e.g. team games, group work	■ Social skills training programme Carefully consider choice of partner/group member Heighten staff awareness	Seek support from school nurse/doctor, child and adolescent mental health service, behavioural support team, educational psychologist
■ Appropriateness of behaviour, e.g. student may hum, tap, fiddle	■ Behaviour management programme Social skills programme Allow student to 'fiddle' with an agreed object, e.g. Blu-Tack®, stress balls Allow student to chew something, e.g. gum	
■ Confidence, self-esteem and self-image	■ Pastoral care/mentoring Facilitate 'circle of friends' scheme Anger/anxiety management programme	
■ Mood swings	■ Heighten staff and peers' awareness	
■ Emotional difficulties, e.g. anxiety, sense of failure, frustration, anger, jealousy	■ Pastoral care/mentoring Self-esteem group at school Facilitate 'circle of friends' scheme	
■ Exaggerated behaviour due to constantly living in stressful situation	■ Provide safe environment for student to discuss issues and have regular contact with adult mentor	■ Refer to Further reading

Occupational Therapy Approaches for Secondary Special Needs © Whurr Publishers Ltd 2002

MC1 **ADD/ADHD**

MC2 Autistic spectrum disorders including Asperger's syndrome

The autistic spectrum disorders cover a broad range of behaviours. The majority of students, seen in mainstream secondary schools, who are diagnosed with an autistic spectrum disorder, are likely to have Asperger's syndrome.

Definition

Asperger's syndrome is an autistic spectrum disorder and individuals with Asperger's syndrome are commonly described as having a triad of impairment in:

- social interaction;
- social communication;
- social imagination.

In order to be given a medical diagnosis of Asperger's syndrome the individual must meet certain diagnostic criteria and be formally assessed by a specialist medical practitioner. The two major diagnostic instruments currently in use by clinicians are the Diagnostic and Statistical Manual of Mental Disorder (DSM IV) and International Classification of Diseases, 10th edition (ICD-10) .

Recent research suggests that one in six children with Asperger's syndrome also have clear signs of attention deficit hyperactivity disorder (Eisenmajer et al. 1996). Children with Asperger's syndrome have also been identified in the population who have disorders of attention, motor control and perception, referred to as DAMP (Attwood 1998)

Cause

The precise cause of this autistic spectrum disorder cannot yet be specified. It is a developmental disorder with several possible causes including genetic fragility and environmental factors, but is not considered to be caused by emotional deprivation or upbringing.

Presenting features

Students with Asperger's syndrome may have some of the following features in varying degrees of severity:

- inappropriate behaviour due to lack of understanding of social rules;
- failure to initiate contact with others;
- lack of empathy;
- lack of spontaneity and flexibility;
- failure to share experiences;
- considered 'odd' by teachers or peers;
- lack of insight of cause and effect;

- superficially perfect expressive but pedantic/stereotypical speech;
- abnormal intonation;
- abnormal/inappropriate use of language;
- literal understanding;
- lack of facial expression;
- abnormal gaze/gesture and 'odd' posturing;
- can be resistant to change;
- difficulty with abstract concepts;

- obsessional interests;
- motor clumsiness;
- problems with attention;
- sensory sensitivity;
- anxiety;
- depression;
- destructive behaviour arising from anger/frustration.

Treatment

No treatment has yet been proved to cure the condition of autistic spectrum disorder. The student may be offered different types of intervention to cope with the non-understandable world. The most common approaches are:

- social skills training;
- behaviour modification;
- sensory modulation;
- manipulation of the environment;
- social stories;
- Treatment and Education of Austistic and Communication Handicapped Children – TEACCH (Schopler et al. 1995)

Prognosis

Although the symptoms may persist, students can learn strategies to help modify their behaviour.

References

Attwood T (1998) Asperger's Syndrome: A Guide for Parents and Professionals. London: Jessica Kingsley.

Eisenmajer R, Prior M, Leekman S, Wing L, Gould J, Welham M, Ong B (1996) Comparison of clinical symptoms in autism and Asperger's syndrome. Journal of the American Academy of Child and Adolescent Psychiatry 35: 1523-1531.

Schopler E, Mesibor GB, Hearsey K (1995) Structured teaching in the TEACCH system, in Schopler E, Mesibor GB (eds) Learning and Cognition in Autism. New York: Plenum Press.

Wing L, Gould J (1979) Severe impairments of social interaction and associated abnormalities in children: epidemiology and classification. Journal of Autism and Childhood Schizophrenia 9(1): 11-29.

Further information

The National Autistic Society Headquarters
393 City Road
London EC1V 1NG
Tel: 020 7833 2299
Fax 020 7833 9666
Email: nas@nas.org.uk
www.nas.org.uk

Further reading

Attwood T (1998) Asperger's Syndrome: A Guide for Parents and Professionals. London: Jessica Kingsley.

Cumine V, Leach J, Stevenson G (1998) Asperger's Syndrome – A Practical Guide for Teachers. London: Fulton.

Grandin T (1995) Thinking in Pictures. New York: Doubleday.

Jones G (2000) Education Provision for Children with Autism and Asperger's Syndrome. London: Fulton.

Jordan R, Jones G (1999) Meeting the Needs of Children with Autistic Spectrum Disorders. London: Fulton.

Leicester City Council and Leicestershire County Council (1998) Asperger Syndrome – Practical Strategies for the Classroom: A Teacher's Guide. London: National Autistic Society.

National Autistic Society (2000) Inclusion and Autism: Is it Working? London. National Autistic Society.

Reed CL (2001) Quick Reference to Occupational Therapy, 2nd edn. Gaithersburg, MD: Aspen Publishers.

Schopler E, Reichler RJ, DeVellis RF, Daily K (1980) Towards objective classification of childhood autism: Childhood Autism Rating Scale. Journal of Autism and Developmental Disorders 10: 91-101.

Smith Myles B, Southwick J (1999) Asperger Syndrome and Difficult Moments. Shawnee Mission, KS: Autism Asperger Publishing Company.

Whitaker P (2001) Challenging Behaviour and Autism: Making Sense – Making Progress. London: National Autistic Society.

Wing L (1998) The Autistic Spectrum: A Guide for Parents and Professionals, 2nd edn. London: National Autistic Society.

Further resources

Social stories – refer to book Asperger's Syndrome by Tony Attwood (1998: 33-35).
Circle of Friends – refer to Asperger's Syndrome by Tony Attwood (1998: 165-166).
Gaining Face – CD Rom for teaching people how to interpret facial expressions, available from the National Autistic Society.
Websites: www.tonyattwood.com,
www.teacch.com

Table 2.2 Autistic spectrum disorder

Students diagnosed with autistic spectrum disorder will present with varying degrees of need depending on the severity of their condition. The presenting features mentioned below are an extensive list and may not all be relevant.

Management should be targeted for the individual student after an analysis of the observed behaviours. It will then be important to decide whether the behaviour needs to be managed or changed. It may be necessary to seek advice from your SENCO in order to implement some of these approaches.

Possible Presenting Features	Management Approaches	Further Advice from SENCO
Behaviour		
■ Tendency towards routines, rituals and obsessions ■ Inappropriate behaviour due to lack of understanding of social rules ■ Difficulty coping with unstructured and/or unfamiliar situations	Behaviour management programme/strategies Social skills training programme Heighten staff and peers, awareness Provide a clear structure and inform student of changes in advance	
■ Does not always respond to sanctions ■ Often off task, distractible and has difficulty sustaining attention	■ Behaviour management programme Set short, attainable goals and give regular breaks Negotiate and agree on a timespan for working on specific tasks, e.g. use timers Limit distractions – only essential items in work area Frequent teacher feedback and redirection Obtain student's attention by using agreed non-verbal cues	Seek advice from advisory team for Asperger's syndrome, child and adolescent mental health service, specialist speech and language therapist, behavioural support team, educational psychologist
■ Inappropriate responses to sensory input – auditory, visual, tactile, taste, smell	■ Heighten staff awareness that student may over- or under-react to 'normal' auditory, visual, tactile, taste, smell, e.g. drill, school bell, telephone, textures, materials	
■ Tendency to interrupt	■ Social skills training programme	
■ Inappropriate movements, e.g. stereotyped movement patterns, hand clapping, rocking	■ Behaviour management programme Social skills training programme	

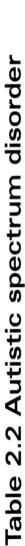

Possible Presenting Features	Management Approaches	Further Advice from SENCO
■ Failure to complete work	■ Clarify expectations, e.g. structured information on what student is to achieve ■ Share schemes of work and syllabus with student so they know exactly what is to be covered in timespan	■ Refer to Appendix (A5)
Physical gross motor skills		**Refer to gross motor co-ordination skill sheet (F1)**
■ Poor or unusual posture, e.g. slouching, tense/rigid	■ Encourage appropriate seating – check table/chair size height	■ Refer to Occupational Therapy sheet (OT1)
■ Rigidity/movements lack fluency ■ Low muscle tone – flopping/propping against objects for support	■ Break down task and practise individual stages ■ Provide a graded fitness programme	■ Refer to James Russell's *Graded Motor Activities*; Elphinston, Pook, *The Core Workout* (see
■ Poor spatial concepts, judging distances and speed	■ Explore alternative PE/games options which can be systematically taught, e.g. gymnastics, swimming, athletics	Further reading) and Occupational Therapy sheet (OT6)
■ Difficulty participating in team games, e.g. interpreting rules, social interaction, varying nature of games, turn-taking	■ Clear and precise explanation of the expectation of the players and rules of the game ■ Explore alternative PE/games options which are more predictable and not team-based	
■ Dislikes physical contact or reduced awareness of physical space	■ Social skills training programme	
Physical fine motor dexterity		**Refer to fine manual dexterity skill sheet (F2) and visual motor integration sheet (F6)**
■ Impaired pen grasp and variable pressure, hampering sustained written output	■ Try alternative writing implements but may need to accept 'awkward' pen grasp and reduced speed of writing ■ Accept that quantity of written work will be reduced goals and set attainable goals	■ Refer to Occupational Therapy sheet (OT3) and Appendix (A2) ■ Refer to Appendices (A1) and (A3)
■ Lack of fluency and neatness of handwriting	■ Consider extra time allowance in exams or adult support as an amanuensts ■ Consider use of alternative recording methods, e.g. dictaphone, word processor, part-prepared worksheets	
■ Poor manipulation of equipment, e.g. scissors, compass	■ Break down task and practise specific skill ■ Improve fine motor co-ordination ■ Trial alternative equipment	■ Refer to educational psychologist ■ Refer to Occupational Therapy sheet (OT5)
■ Difficulty sharing equipment	■ Explain which items are to be shared by whom	■ Refer to Equipment resources (ER)

Occupational Therapy Approaches for Secondary Special Needs © Whurr Publishers Ltd 2002

MC2 ASD (continued)

Table 2.2 Autistic spectrum disorder

52

Possible Presenting Features	Management Approaches	Further Advice from SENCO
Organizational		**Refer to organizational skills sheet (F3)**
■ Finding way around school	■ Practise route to new classrooms/subject areas prior to commencing each new school year To miss crowded corridors, students may be allowed to leave early, appropriately supervised	
■ Poor ability to organize self and task unaware of expectations misconstrues the meaning of instructions limited problem-solving skills	■ Give clear expectations and ensure student understands them, e.g. work schedules Break down task and set attainable goals Use strategies, e.g. personal timetable, schedules, checklists, calenders, pictorial clues	■ Refer to Appendix (**A5**) ■ Refer to Occupational Therapy sheet (**OT7**)
■ Reduced concept of time	■ Teach coping strategies, e.g. use alarms on watches, timer, timed checklists	
■ Inappropriate sense of danger/no sense of danger	■ Raise the student's awareness of danger Heighten staff awareness and undertake risk assessment if appropriate Paired working/adult support Consider use of safety checklists Adult monitoring in unstructured situations	■ Refer to school health and safety policy
■ Inability to generalize skills into unfamiliar situations	■ Heighten staff awareness	
■ Difficulty managing equipment, material, books, etc. needed for school day	■ Provide secure, accessible locker space	■ Refer to Occupational Therapy sheet (**OT7**)

Possible Presenting Features

Communication

Receptive language
- interprets literally what is said
- misunderstands intent of word with multiple meanings
- difficulty with abstract concepts
- difficulty following instructions

Expressive language
- tendency to talk on one topic
- interrupts/talks over others, difficulty with turn-taking
- makes irrelevant comments

- Uses language well but has difficulty adjusting it to a social context
- Difficulty recognizing subtleties of language

- Inability to associate emotion with spoken word or facial expression

Writing skills
- difficulty with creative and abstract thought
- keeping to topic

- logical organization of work

- Incomplete work

Management Approaches

- Slowly give unambiguous instructions
  Check that student has understood your instructions
  Clarify words which have double meaning and explain metaphors
  Encourage student to ask for clarification when necessary
  Ensure verbal information is limited to the amount a student can manage
  When presenting new concepts and abstract material be as concrete as possible
  Use written/pictorial support as appropriate

- Social use of language programme
  Facilitate 'circle of friends' scheme

- Use available materials, e.g. 'Gaining Faces' CD Rom (See Further resources in this section)

- Give guidelines for creative writing
  Use writing frames to structure work
  Clearly define expectations of task
  Encourage student to pre-plan content of work

- Use mind mapping
  Use cue cards identifying stages

- Use home/school record so parent is aware of homework requirements and ensure student fully understands expectations of the task
  Discuss reason with student and parent
  Set time limit for task

Further Advice from SENCO

Refer to auditory processing and memory skill sheet (F12)

- Seek advice from advisory team for Asperger's syndrome or specialist provision, specialist speech and language therapist

- Refer to Appendix (A5)

- Refer to Further reading

- Seek advice from advisory team for Asperger's syndrome, specialist speech therapist and language therapist, occupational therapist

- Refer to Further reading

Table 2.2 Autistic spectrum disorders

Possible Presenting Features	Management Approaches	Further Advice from SENCO
Self-care		
■ Difficulty in daily living tasks slow at dressing, difficulty with fastenings, dishevelled use of cutlery general appearance	■ Social skills/life training programme Allow extra time to complete activity, e.g. PE changing Adapt fastenings, discuss with parents and student the possibility of wearing alternative clothing, e.g. polo shirts	■ Seek further advise from occupational therapist, child and adolescent mental health service
handling money	Ensure lunchtime staff are aware of student's difficulty	
standing in lunch queue	Stand at front/back of queue or go early for lunch	
■ Reluctance to undertake personal hygiene routines, e.g. toileting due to ritual obsessions	■ Behaviour management programme Social skills training programme	■ Seek advice from clinical psychologist, school nurse, school doctor
■ 'Faddy' eater leading to restricted diet	■ Discuss with parents. Encourage a balanced diet	■ Seek advice from dietician
Social, emotional and psychological		**Refer to social interaction skill sheet (F13)**
■ Anxiety, depression, anger, frustration due to constantly living in stressful situation Becomes stressed due to inflexibility Inflexible thinking – no idea there may be two sides to a dilemma Often unable to tolerate making a mistake Emotional immaturity, naive and often lacks tact Problems forming and maintaining relationships Reduced or inappropriate eye contact Reduced awareness of personal space Poor self-esteem Difficulty demonstrating empathy and expressing emotions Treat all people equally even strangers Can have high pain threshold Feelings of persecution Difficulty with separating fact from opinion, shades of grey	■ Choose tutor group carefully Heighten staff awareness in all subject areas Pastoral care/mentoring Provide opportunity for daily contact with tutor/SENCO to check attendance/homework etc. Social skills training programme Ensure as much structure is in place as possible Facilitate 'circle of friends' scheme, (refer to Further reading) Choose peers carefully when planning group work	Seek further advice from advisory team for Asperger's syndrome or specialist provision, child and adolescent mental health service, speech and language therapist

Occupational Therapy Approaches for Secondary Special Needs © Whurr Publishers Ltd 2002

Cerebral palsy

Definition

Cerebral palsy is a disorder of posture and movement.

Cause

Cerebral palsy is caused by damage to the brain before, during or after birth while the brain is still developing. In many cases there is no obvious cause.

Classification

There are three types of cerebral palsy, depending on which part of the brain is damaged – spastic, athetoid and ataxic. Many people with cerebral palsy have a combination of two or more types and may have additional complications/ diagnoses such as epilepsy which are usually well controlled with medication.

The complexity of cerebral palsy and its effects vary from one person to another, as do the parts of the body which can be affected:

hemiplegia – when one side of the body is affected;

diplegia – when both legs are affected but the arms are less affected;

quadriplegia – total body involvement, including oral difficulties.

Spastic cerebral palsy

Spastic cerebral palsy increases the tone in muscle groups, which results in tightness in the muscles and reduced range of movement in joints. This makes fluent and co-ordinated movement very difficult. This tightness or stiffness, which can be increased by strenuous activity and excitation, is always present so a person with spastic cerebral palsy has to work harder than his or her peers when walking or moving.

Athetoid cerebral palsy

Students with this kind of cerebral palsy make involuntary movements because their muscles rapidly change from floppy to tense in a way that they cannot control. They find it hard to maintain balance and postures as movement in one part of the body influences control and posture in the rest of the body. Their speech may be hard to understand because they have difficulty controlling their tongue, breathing and vocal cords. Hearing problems are common.

Ataxic cerebral palsy

Ataxia affects the whole body causing jerky, uncontrolled movements. Students with this kind of cerebral palsy find it very hard to balance, may have poor spatial awareness and are generally uncoordinated. Usually a student will be able to walk, but will probably be very unsteady. They may also have shaky hand movements, jerky eye movements and laboured speech.

Presenting features

Cerebral palsy is a condition that affects movement in varying forms and with varying degrees of severity. No two people with cerebral palsy are the same. Some students are barely affected whilst others will have difficulty talking, walking, using their hands and sitting without support. In some cases the student will need help with everyday functional tasks, e.g. toileting, dressing, eating.

Many students with cerebral palsy may have some of the following features, in varying degrees of severity:

1 Gross motor

- stiffness in joints;
- muscle weakness;
- spasms in muscle/increased tone;
- reduced stamina/fatigue with little reserves of energy;
- slow, awkward or jerky movements;
- activity of one movement often results in unwanted movements in another part of the body;
- poor balance in sitting or standing;
- uncoordinated walking pattern;
- use of frame, stick or crutches for mobility;
- wheelchair-dependent.

2 Fine motor

- abrupt, jerky hand movements;
- tightness of upper limb(s);
- weakness in muscles;
- spasm in muscles;
- poor manipulative skills;
- poor self-help skills;
- difficulty with eye–hand co-ordination;
- difficulty with using both hands together.

3 Perception

- poor memory skills;
- reduced concentration/easily distracted from task;
- underdeveloped or disordered visual perceptual skills;
- disturbed sensory perception;
- impaired visual/auditory skills.

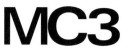

4 Social/emotional factors

- reduced concentration
- low self-esteem;
- learnt dependency;
- anxiety and frustration;
- indistinct speech;
- difficulty coming to terms with disability;
- difficulty establishing relationships with peer group.

Many students with cerebral palsy have average or above-average intelligence. Some students do have general learning difficulties, which may be mild, moderate or severe. Students with cerebral palsy may have a 'specific learning difficulty' because a particular part of their brain has been affected.

Treatment

There is no cure for cerebral palsy, but the student may be offered different types of intervention to help their physical and emotional development:

- physiotherapy including hydrotherapy;
- occupational therapy;
- speech and language therapy;
- medication to control muscle spasm;
- orthopaedic intervention/splints/surgery;
- counselling/emotional support.

Prognosis

Cerebral palsy is not a progressive condition. However, without the correct therapy and family support, the student's ability to maintain walking and movement may be compromised resulting in deterioration. Some difficulties intensify as functional demands increase at home, in school and in the wider community. As students get older with an increase in height and weight, their physical skills may decrease, e.g. a student who was walking may need to use a wheelchair for some or all of the time. The hormonal changes of adolescence combined with the heightened awareness of their physical disability may affect their motivation and desire for independence.

Further information

SCOPE
6 Market Road
London WN7 0PW
Tel: 020 7619 7100
Email: cphelpline@scope.org.uk
www.scope.org.uk

Cerebral Palsy Helpline
PO Box 833
Milton Keynes
Buckinghamshire MK12 5NY
Tel: 0808 8003333
Email: cphelpline@scope.org.uk
www.scope.org.uk

Hemi Helpline
Bedford House
215 Balham High Street
London
SW17 7BQ
Tel: 020 8767 0210
Email: support@hemihelp.org.uk
www.hemihelp.org.uk
Information on aids and communication

The Bobath Centre
250 East End Road
London
N2 8AU
Tel: 0120 8444 3355
Email: info@bobathlondon.co.uk
www.bobath.org.uk

Bobath Scotland
2028 Great Western Road
Glasgow
G13 2HA
Tel: 0141 950 2922
Email: info@bobathscotland.org.uk
www.bobathscotland.org.uk

Bobath Children's Therapy Centre, Wales
19 Park Road
Whitchurch
Cardiff
CF4 7BP
Tel: 02920 522600
Email: bobathwales@ukgateway.net
www.bobathwales.co.uk

ACE (Aiding Communication in Education)
Centre Advisory Trust
92 Windmill Road
Headington
Oxford OX3 7DR
Tel: 01865 759800
Email: info@ace-centre.org.uk
www.ace-centre.org.uk

ACE Centre Advisory Trust - North
1 Broadbent Road
Watersheddings
Oldham
OL1 4HU
Tel: 0161 6271358
Email: ace-north@ace-north.org
www.ace-centre.org.uk

CALL Centre
University of Edinburgh
Patterson's Land
Hollyrood Road
Edinburgh
EH8 8AQ
Tel: 0131 6516236
Email: call.centre@ed.ac.uk
www.callcentrescotland.org.uk

See also information communication technology checklist (Appendix **A3**).

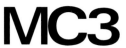

Further reading

Cogher L, Savage E, Smith M (1992) Cerebral Palsy: The Child and Young Person. London: Chapman and Hall.

Geralis E (1998) Children with Cerebral Palsy – A Parent's Guide, 2nd edn. Bethesda, MD: Woodbine House.

Miller F, Bachrach SJ (1995) Cerebral Palsy – A Complete Guide to Caregiving. Baltimore, MD: The Johns Hopkins University Press.

Pickles P (1998) Managing Curriculum for Children with Severe Motor Difficulties: A Practical Approach. London: Fulton.

Reed CL. (2001) Quick Reference to Occupational Therapy, 2nd edn. Baltimore, MD: Aspen Publishers.

Willner L (1996) Getting on with Cerebral Palsy – From Adolescence to Old Age. London: Scope.

Wilson C, Jade R (1999) Whose Voice is it Anyway? Talking to Disabled Young People at School. London: Alliance for Inclusive Education.

Guidelines for Teachers booklets are available from Hemi Help – No. 2 The Student with Hemiplegia in Secondary Education.

Further resources

Don't Give Up – Growing Up with Hemiplegia - a video by children for children, available from Hemi Help.

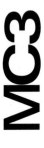

MC3

Table 2.3 Cerebral palsy, including hemiplegia and diplegia

It is essential that

1 **A risk assessment is carried out prior to the student entering school and repeated in accordance with the school or county manual handling policy**
2 **Staff receive regular training in manual handling in accordance with the manual handling policy**
3 **Staff liaise with the physiotherapist/occupational therapist since inappropriate activities may lead to increased problems and/or injury**

Students diagnosed with cerebral palsy will present with varying areas of need depending on the severity of their condition. The presenting features mentioned below are an extensive list and may not all be relevant.

Management should be targeted for the individual student. It may be necessary to seek advice from the SENCO in order to implement some of these approaches.

Possible Presenting Features	Management Approaches	Further Advice via SENCO
Health – depending on type and severity of condition		**Refer to gross motor coordination skill sheet (F1) and fine manual dexterity skill sheets (F2)**
■ Increased weight due to immobility	■ Undertake risk assessment Heighten awareness e.g. of peers and staff Implications for manual handling, therefore use hoist Monitor dietary intake in discussion with family	■ Refer to school health and safety policy ■ Seek advice from school nurse, doctor
■ Postural deformities, e.g. trunk, hips, feet, upper limbs	■ Ensure correct seating is available and used If student has splints, liaise with physiotherapist Ensure physiotherapy programme is timetabled	■ Seek advice from physiotherapist, occupational therapist
■ Reduced ability to move joints – pain increases on activity	■ Regular physiotherapy programme as directed by the physiotherapist Use prescribed splints	
■ Time out of school for hospital appointments, e.g. surgery, physiotherapy	■ Discuss strategies with parents and student to ensure missed work is passed on to student Arrange home tutor if required	

Possible Presenting Features	Management Approaches	Further Advice via SENCO
Physical		
■ Mobility reduced mobility sometimes resulting in use of wheelchair/walking frame/crutches reduced stamina poor spatial awareness	■ When planning timetable consider close proximity of classroom and minimize use of stairs Discuss use of wheelchair for transit between lessons Check all equipment is available in school and duplicate if necessary Adult support around school Consider student being the first person in and out of classroom to minimize risk of accidents Provide locker to reduce need to carry equipment Limit amount of walking around the classroom/laboratory Use backpack or diagonal strap bag to keep hands free	■ Discuss with person responsible for timetable planning Seek advice from physiotherapist, wheelchair service, occupational therapist, advisory teacher
■ Difficulty participating in PE/games	■ Discuss with student and physiotherapist PE/games options that are appropriate and attainable to ensure self-esteem is maintained	
■ Timetabling for physiotherapy exercises	■ Provide room and privacy for therapy Ensure necessary equipment is available, including hoist Discuss with student, parents and physiotherapist suitable time and exercise regime	■ Refer to school manual handling policy and undertake risk assessment Seek advice from advisory teacher
■ Poor posture affecting functional performance in sitting/standing	■ Check chair/wheelchair height in relation to working surfaces especially for practical subjects Ensure supportive seating is available, e.g. perching stool	■ Refer to Occupational Therapy sheet (**OT1**) Seek advice from occupational therapist, wheelchair service
■ Access into buildings including classrooms, toilets, showers, library, canteen	■ Check height/numbers of steps/stairs and consider ramps/rails Check positions of doors and handles and alter if necessary Consider the need/viability of stair climbers Look at space in rooms – toilet, showers, etc. and consider rearranging furniture Consider the need for structural alteration, e.g. viability of lifts, extensions	■ Seek advice from physiotherapists, advisory teachers, occupational therapist, manual handling advisor, county surveyor
around external school facilities	■ Consider the need for ramps/rails or alternative route around site	■ Seek advice from occupational therapist, advisory teacher, county surveyor

Occupational Therapy Approaches for Secondary Special Needs © Whurr Publishers Ltd 2002

MC3 CP (continued)

Table 2.3 Cerebral palsy

Possible Presenting Features	Management Approaches	Further Advice via SENCO
Physical (continued)		
■ Transport – travelling safely to and from school	■ Use of appropriate transport, e.g. rails/ramps/seat belts/safety harness/wheelchair clamps Appropriate seating/wheelchair which meets LEA safety requirements	■ Refer to LEA Transport Department Seek advice from occupational therapist, physiotherapist, wheelchair services
■ School trips/field trips – access mobility and transport	■ Use of appropriate transport, e.g. lift on bus/coach/wheelchair clamps Portaramps or fixed ramps may be requested Pre-check access and facilities, e.g. toilet, dining area, parking area Ensure appropriate equipment available – extra support may be needed Arrange suitable transport so student can safely travel as part of the group Consider appropriateness of venue and seek alternatives if needed	■ Refer to school trips policy
■ Fine motor reduced manual dexterity leading to lack of accuracy when handling instruments/materials in practical lessons	■ Check student is in optimum position for function, e.g. elbows supported Trial alternative instruments/tools and check appropriate equipment is available. Consider buddy/adult support	■ Refer to Occupational Therapy sheet (**OT1**) ■ Refer to Equipment resources (**ER**) Seek advice from occupational therapist, advisory teachers
poor written skills, e.g. presentation of work, stamina, speed of writing	■ Check student is in optimum position for function Use an angled surface Use alternative methods of recording, e.g. part prepared worksheets, photocopied sheets, word processor Consider adult support	■ Refer to Occupational Therapy sheet (**OT1**) ■ Refer to Appendix (**A1**)
accessing ICT equipment	■ Investigate alternative ICT equipment, e.g. switches, key guard, mouse	■ Seek advice from ICT advisor Refer to Appendix (**A3**)

Occupational Therapy Approaches for Secondary Special Needs © Whurr Publishers Ltd 2002

MC3 CP (continued)

Possible Presenting Features	Management Approaches	Further Advice via SENCO
Self-care	**Privacy is paramount – discuss with student and parents**	
■ Toilet – access and transfers	■ Undertake risk assessment Ensure adequate space for wheelchair, student and helper Consider rails, hoist, changing table	■ Refer to school manual handling policy Seek further advice from physiotherapist, occupational therapist, advisory teachers, manual handling advisor
■ Self-catherization	■ Provide privacy Identify safe and efficient methods Provide adapted equipment, e.g. toilet chair	■ Seek advice from school nurse
■ Showering – access and transfers	■ Undertake risk assessment Ensure adequate space for wheelchair, student and helper Consider the need for supportive equipment, e.g. shower chair, rails	■ Refer to school manual handling policy Seek advice from occupational therapist
■ Slow at dressing/managing clothing/fastenings	■ Practise dressing skills and allocate time for this. Discuss with student/parent adapting clothing/fastenings, e.g. skirts/trousers with elasticated waist, attach loops on waistbands to help pull up skirt/trousers/pants, velcro fastenings. Allow extra time Provide adult help	■ Seek advice from occupational therapist
■ Mealtimes mobility and adequate space around dining hall	■ Ensure clear pathways to allow for wheelchair manoeuvrability Position student at end of table with friends	
obtaining meal from serving hatch/carrying tray	■ Trial of alternative trays Meal collected by friend or adult	■ Refer to Equipment resources (**ER**)
use of cup/cutlery	■ Provision of appropriate cutlery, cups, plate guards, non-slip mats following discussion with student/parent	■ Seek advice from occupational therapist
■ Organization having correct equipment available carrying books, bags, equipment around school	■ Provide easily accessible and secure locker Use back pack/diagonal bag/bag on wheelchair Consider buddy support	

Occupational Therapy Approaches for Secondary Special Needs © Whurr Publishers Ltd 2002

MC3 CP (continued)

Table 2.3 Cerebral palsy

Possible Presenting Features	Management Approaches	Further Advice via SENCO
Perception		**Refer to brief introduction to perception (F4) and vision and ocular motor control skill sheet (F5)**
■ Visual perception – interpreting visual information figure ground discrimination, e.g. finding place on board/page spatial awareness, e.g. directionality visual closure, e.g. visualization of processes such as lifecycles in biology	■ Refer to visual figure ground discrimination skill sheet (F9) Refer to visual spatial relationships skill sheet (F7) Refer to visual closure skill sheet (F10)	
■ Vision and ocular motor control difficulty keeping focus on teacher	■ Sit centrally in class facing front	■ Seek advice from occupational therapist, behavioural optometrist
copying from board	Give individual paper e.g. copy of instructions/work written on board	
following text in book/paper	Use reading guide or ruler below line of print/figures in columns	
making directional changes quickly	Expect less fluency in PE activities which require continual turning/visual checking (team games)	
fuzzy/blurred print	Consider use of individual coloured overlays	■ Refer to Appendix (A4)
Communication		
■ Slow and laboured speech	■ Heighten teachers' and peers' awareness of student's difficulty Allow extra time for student to respond	■ Seek advice from speech and language therapist
■ Poor clarity of speech	Allow student to finish sentence without interrupting flow	
■ Little or no understandable speech	■ Implement use of communication aid as directed by speech and language therapist	
■ Slow at processing receptive language	■ Allow extra time for student to process	
■ Difficulty with physical expression (non-verbal communication)	■ Heighten teachers' and peers' awareness Heighten student's awareness	

Occupational Therapy Approaches for Secondary Special Needs © Whurr Publishers Ltd 2002

MC3 CP (continued)

Possible Presenting Features	Management Approaches	Further Advice via SENCO
Social, emotional and psychological		**Refer to social interaction skill sheet (F13)**
■ Poor self-concept and low self-esteem, feelings of being different	■ Provide pastoral support Choose peers carefully when planning group work Provide frequent opportunities for student to experience success Increase staff awareness Provide opportunities to meet with other disabled young people to share experiences	■ Seek advice from child and adolescent mental health service, educational psychologist
■ Frustrated due to lack of ability	■ Set attainable goals and adapt activity to enhance success Consider buddy working – choose buddy carefully Provide pastoral support	
■ Depression due to awareness of own physical limitations	■ Provide pastoral support Discuss concerns with parents Seek professional counselling support for student	

MC4 Developmental co-ordination disorder including dyspraxia

Definition

Developmental co-ordination disorder is a marked impairment in the development of motor co-ordination which significantly interferes with academic achievement or activities of daily living.

In order to be given a medical diagnosis of developmental co-ordination disorder the student must meet certain criteria as outlined in the Diagnostic and Statistical Manual of Mental Disorders (DSM IV) or International Classification of Diseases, 10th edition (ICD10) called specific developmental disorder of motor function.

Developmental co-ordination disorder is the current term now commonly used to describe students with motor co-ordination difficulties. It has also been known as perceptual motor dysfunction, clumsy child syndrome, minimal brain dysfunction or motor learning difficulty. It is an umbrella term which includes developmental dyspraxia (difficulty with motor planning), sensory integrative dysfunction and DAMP (this is a combination of developmental co-ordination disorder and attention deficit hyperactivity disorder as there are deficits in attention, motor control and perception).

Cause

The exact cause is currently unknown.

Presenting features

The manifestations of this disorder vary with age and development. For example, younger children may display clumsiness and delays in achieving developmental milestones (e.g. walking, crawling, sitting, tying shoe laces, buttoning shirts, zipping trousers). Older children may display difficulties with the motor aspects of assembling puzzles, building models, playing ball, manipulating equipment, drawing and handwriting.

Students' skill development is impaired so they are unable to perform some tasks at an age-appropriate level. This often labels them as clumsy or inefficient and they may be unable to transfer skills to similar tasks.

Students with developmental co-ordination disorder may have some of the following features in varying degrees of severity:

1   Gross motor

- falls, trips and bumps into things;
- looks awkward when walking, running, hopping, skipping;
- difficulty co-ordinating and maintaining swimming strokes/PE activities;
- lacks stamina/seeks support;
- low quality muscle tone and seems weak;

Occupational Therapy Approaches for Secondary Special Needs © Whurr Publishers Ltd 2002

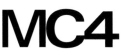
- difficulty with ball games;
- difficulty planning and carrying out a sequence of movements.

2 Fine motor

- difficulty with all pen and paper tasks;
- poor fine motor co-ordination, manipulation and dexterity;
- poor manipulation of tools, e.g. scissors, rulers, compass;
- reduced speed for fine motor tasks and impaired quality of finished work.

3 Organization

- difficulty generalizing learnt skills to other areas;
- difficulty planning and carrying out a sequence of movements both gross and fine;
- poor organization of self, and within own environment;
- poor sequencing and timing skills;
- difficulty with problem solving;
- spatial/perceptual difficulties;
- poor self-care skills, e.g. untidy appearance.

4 Social/emotional factors

- lack confidence;
- be the class clown or withdrawn;
- have awareness of difficulties leading to low self-esteem;
- exhibit adult dependency – 'learnt helplessness';
- have learnt failure therefore unwilling to try;
- be immature;
- have difficulty making friends;
- be distractible – difficulty sustaining attention;
- show inappropriate responses to sensory stimuli – auditory, visual or tactile;
- suffer frustration – understands end task but cannot plan how to get there;
- have difficulty establishing relationships with peers.

Treatment

The student may be offered different types of intervention depending on local policies and availability of resources:

- occupational therapy;
- physiotherapy;
- speech and language therapy;

- child and adolescent mental health service;
- behavioural support team.

Prognosis

Developmental co-ordination disorder is not progressive; it does not become more severe as the child becomes older. However some difficulties may become more apparent as functional demands at home, in school and in the wider community increase. In some cases lack of co-ordination continues through adolescence and adulthood.

Further information

Dyspraxia Foundation
8 West Alley
Hitchin
Hertfordshire SG5 1EG
Administration tel: 01462 455016; helpline tel: 01462 454986
Email: admin@dyspraxiafoundation.org.uk
www: dyspraxiafoundation.org.uk

Further reading

Chu S (1995) Children with Developmental Dyspraxia – Information for Parents and Teachers. Hitchin: Dyspraxia Foundation.

Chu S (1998a) Developmental dyspraxia 1: the diagnosis. British Journal of Therapy and Rehabilitation 5(3): 131-38.

Chu S (1998b) Developmental dyspraxia 2: evaluation and treatment. British Journal of Therapy and Rehabilitation 5(4): 176-80.

Kirby A (1999) Dyspraxia – The Hidden Handicap. London: Souvenir Press.

Kranowitz CS (1998) The Out-of-sync Child: Recognizing and Coping with Sensory Integration Dysfunction. New York: Pedigree Book.

McKinley I, Gordon N (1980) Helping Clumsy Children. Edinburgh: Churchill Livingstone.

Parkin S, Padley M. Working With Clumsy Children. A Practical Approach For Teachers. Available from Bannerdale Centre, Bannerdale Road, Sheffield S7 2EW Tel: 0114 2506842.

Penso DE (1993) Perceptuo-motor Difficulties. Theory and Strategies to Help Children, Adolescents and Adults. London: Chapman and Hall.

Praxis Makes Perfect and Praxis Makes Perfect 2 - available from the Dyspraxia Foundation.

Reed CL (2001) Quick Reference to Occupational Therapy, 2nd edn. Baltimore, MD: Aspen Publishers.

Ripley K (2001) Inclusion for Children with Dyspraxia/DCD. London: Fulton.

Ripley K, Daines B, Barrett J (1997) Dyspraxia – A Guide for Teachers and Parents. London: Fulton.

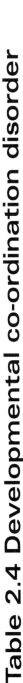

MC4

Table 2.4 Developmental co-ordination disorder

Students diagnosed with developmental co-ordination disorder will present with varying degrees of need depending on the severity of their condition. The presenting features mentioned below are an extensive list and may not all be relevant.

Management should be targeted for the individual student. It may be necessary to seek advice from your SENCO in order to implement some of these approaches.

Possible Presenting Features	Management Approaches	Further Advice via SENCO
Students may be reluctant to take part in activities due to anticipated difficulties based on past failure		**Refer to gross motor co-ordination skill sheet (F1)**
Physical gross motor skills		

■ Low muscle tone
  reduced stamina and fatigue
  'earthbound', lacks balance
  propping or flopping between activities
  flexible in joints but lacks strength
  difficulty maintaining postures against gravity
	■ Ensure a supported functional posture is used
	  Where possible minimize amount of time required to stand
	  Practise graded motor activities
	  Heighten staff awareness of the effects of low tone on student's performance
		■ Refer to physiotherapist, occupational therapist
		
		■ Refer to Further reading
		  Refer to Occupational Therapy sheet (**OT6**)

■ Co-ordination/balance
  lacks fluency of movements
  appears awkward and uncoordinated
  difficulty executing precise, controlled movements
  lacks the control to sustain balance postures
	■ Carefully graded programme to improve balance
	  Heighten staff awareness of the effects of instability on student's performance
	  Ensure adequate space in work area
	  Check sitting posture is correct and monitored frequently
		■ Refer to physiotherapist, occupational therapist

■ Bilateral skills
  difficulty co-ordinating movements, requiring the use of both sides of the body, e.g. swimming, cycling, playing musical instruments
	■ Break down activity and practise individual component parts
	  Encourage using both hands to establish a bilateral working pattern
		■ Refer to Occupational Therapy sheet (**OT1**)

■ Sequencing and organizing movements
  moving around school
  planning tasks
  ability to anticipate, plan and respond whilst participating in any activity
	■ Encourage student to pre-plan task
	  Provide verbal and physical prompts and reduce amount of prompts as student's abilities improve
	  Heighten staff awareness to importance of giving clear, detailed yet concise instructions
		■ Refer to Occupational Therapy sheet (**OT7**)

MC4

Table 2.4 Developmental co-ordination disorder

Possible Presenting Features	Management Approaches	Further Advice via SENCO
Physical (continued)		

■ Proprioception
  excessive movement/fidgety in an attempt to raise own body awareness
  lacks smooth, controlled movements
  unable to negotiate own body through space
  inability to sustain correct posture
	■ Increase body awareness through graded resisted activities	■ Seek advice from physiotherapist/occupational therapist

■ Reduced sense of danger	■ Heighten awareness of safety issues and undertake health and safety risk assessment	■ Refer to school health and safety policy
Physical fine motor dexterity		**Refer to fine manual dexterity sheet (F2) and visual motor integration (F6)**

■ Reduced manipulative skills effecting all practical tasks	■ Use of alternative/adapted equipment
	  Buddy/adult support
	  Improve manipulative skills through a fine motor programme
		■ Seek further advice from occupational therapist or advisory teachers
		■ Refer to Occupational Therapy sheet (**OT5**)

■ Handwriting
  illegible script
  poor letter formation, spacing and positioning
  untidy due to excessive crossing out and correcting
  variable pressure on writing tool
  reduced quantity of output
  difficulty with creative writing
  not fully established as an automatic skill
	■ Consider alternative recording methods, e.g. ICT, part-prepared worksheets
	  Teach touch-typing and provide regular daily practice
	  Teach study skills – mind mapping, writing frames
	  Set realistic targets
		■ Refer to Appendices (**A1**, **A2** and **A3**)
		■ Refer to Further reading
		■ Refer to Occupational Therapy sheets (**OT3** and **OT4**)

■ Impaired grasp on tools	■ Heighten staff awareness that impaired grasp will affect quality of performance Use adapted equipment/utensils	■ Refer to Occupational Therapy sheets (**OT5**) ■ Refer to Equipment resources sheet (**ER**)

Occupational Therapy Approaches for Secondary Special Needs © Whurr Publishers Ltd 2002

MC4 DCD (continued)

Possible Presenting Features	Management Approaches	Further Advice via SENCO
Physical (continued)		
■ Slow execution of task due to inconsistent hand dominance in practical tasks	■ Allow extra time for completion of task Use part-prepared work Set realistic attainable goals Use buddy/adult support	■ Refer to Appendix (**A5**)
■ Reduced proprioception and tactile awareness resulting in awkward hand function	■ Allow more time for tasks	
Organizational		**Refer to organizational skill sheet (F3)**
■ Organizing self for daily programme and orientation around school building	■ Provide colour-coded timetables Liaise with family/carers regarding consistent strategies to help develop routine	■ Refer to Occupational Therapy sheet (**OT7**)
■ Organizing equipment in preparation for tasks	■ Provide checklists/cue cards identifying required equipment Use cue cards Encourage an uncluttered work space	
■ Inability and lack of awareness to break down components of task when problem solving	■ Use cue cards Give clear, concise, step by step instructions Use task analysis approach Give checklists and reduce prompts as student masters skill	
■ Difficulty in formulating a plan of action when attempting new task	■ Talk through ideas by presenting a variety of scenarios Discuss and identify component parts Give written plan as well as verbal instructions Formulate a plan of action	

MC4

Table 2.4 Developmental co-ordination disorder

Possible Presenting Features	Management Approaches	Further Advice via SENCO
Organizational (continued)		
■ Difficulty coping with changes in routine	■ Talk to student about forthcoming changes to work out strategies Rehearse changed routines, e.g. how to get to new location in advance	■ Refer to school health and safety policy
■ Inappropriate sense of danger and perception of own abilities	■ Heighten staff awareness Raise student's awareness of their skill level Paired working and/or adult support	
■ Incomplete homework	■ Discuss reason with student and parent Consider attending homework club Set realistic goals	
■ Reduced time concept	■ Teach coping strategies, e.g. use alarms, watches, timers, timed checklist/weekly timetable	
■ Inability to generalize skills	■ Heighten staff awareness Use checklists Break down task and work on specific skill areas then link them with similar tasks	
Communication		**Refer to auditory processing and memory skill sheet (F12)**
■ Following, remembering and processing verbal instructions	■ Give clear, concise instructions in small steps, ensure verbal information is limited to amount student can manage Give instructions and allow student to verbalize back to check that he or she has heard and understood Withdraw student to quiet area and give instructions Reinforce with written notes/diagrammatic prompts	■ Seek advice from speech and language therapist, educational psychologist
■ Jumbled thoughts when speaking/writing	■ Heighten student and staff awareness of the difficulty Make notes/underline key points and sequence points prior to writing Encourage student to stop and think before speaking Teach mind-mapping techniques	■ Refer to Further reading

MC4 DCD (continued)

Possible Presenting Features	Management Approaches	Further Advice via SENCO
Communication (continued)		

■ Auditory
  processing the spoken word
  identifying relevant information through background noises
  understanding and responding to instructions
	■ Speak slower and use simple phrases
	  Ask student to speak back instructions
	  Eliminate unnecessary background noises
	  Allow extra time when communicating with student
	  Provide cue cards to support spoken word	

Perception		**Refer to a brief introduction to perception (F4) and vision and ocular motor skill sheet (F5)**

■ Visual perception – interpreting visual information
  figure ground discrimination, e.g. finding place on board/page
  spatial awareness, e.g. directionality
  visual closure, e.g. visualization of processes such as lifecycles in biology
	■ Refer to visual figure ground discrimination skill sheet (**F9**)
	  Refer to visual spatial relationships skill sheet (**F7**)
	  Refer to visual closure skill sheet (**F10**)	

■ Vision and ocular motor control
  difficulty keeping focus on teacher/board
  copying from board
  following text in book/paper
  making directional changes quickly
  fuzzy/blurred print
	■ Sit centrally in class facing front
	  Give individual paper copy of instructions/work written on board
	  Use reading guide or ruler below line of print/figures in columns
	  Expect less fluency in PE activities which require continual turning/visual checking (team games)
	  Consider use of individual coloured overlays
		■ Seek advice from occupational therapist, behavioural optometrist
		
		■ Refer to Appendix (**A4**)

Self-care		

■ Dressing
  small fastenings, laces, zips
  orientation of clothes (inside out and back to front)
  tying tie
 	
  general presentation – dishevelled appearance
	■ Allow extra time when changing/showering for PE
	  Use alternative fastenings, e.g. velcro, elastic laces, elasticated tie
	  Discuss with parents and student the possibility of wearing alternative clothing, e.g. polo shirts, elasticated waist on trousers
	  Remind student to check appearance after changing	

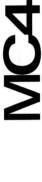

Table 2.4 Developmental co-ordination disorder

Possible Presenting Features	Management Approaches	Further Advice via SENCO
Self-care (continued)		
■ Eating using cutlery difficulty opening packets, yogurt tops, etc. messy, spills food down shirt	■ Advise students to choose canteen food which is easy to cut Suggest provision of a packed lunch Check appearance following a meal	
■ Handling money	■ Ensure lunchtime staff are aware of difficulties	
Social, emotional and psychological		**Refer to social interaction sheet (F13)**
■ Low confidence/poor self-esteem shyness, isolation from peers unwillingness to volunteer for tasks establish strategies to avoid difficult tasks, e.g. sharpening pencil, going out to toilet, clowning about	■ Heighten awareness of staff to difficulties Provide frequent opportunities for students to experience success and personal improvements, not always in relation to others Set realistic, attainable goals Choose peers carefully when planning group work Provide pastoral support/use 'Circle of Friends' scheme Break down and practise component parts of task Feedback to student when clowning strategies are used Behavioural management programme	■ Seek advice from child and adolescent mental health service
■ Prefers company of younger peers or adults	■ Use 'Circle of Friends' scheme Social skills training programme	■ Refer to Further reading
■ Difficulty reading non-verbal cues and emotional expressions	■ Social skills training programme	■ Refer to Further reading

Possible Presenting Features	Management Approaches	Further Advice via SENCO
Social, emotional and psychological (continued)		
■ Frustration, anger and depression, possibly due to awareness of own limitations	■ Provide counselling/pastoral support	■ Seek advice from child and adolescent mental health service, educational psychologist
■ Discrepancy between cognitive ability and performance skills	■ Provide alternative means of recording, e.g. allow use of computer for homework or an adult to scribe Selective paired working to maximize and reinforce areas of strength	■ Refer to Appendices (**A1** and **A3**)
■ Emotionally labile and easily hurt	■ Social skills training programme Pastoral support	

MC5 Dystrophies and degenerative conditions

There are a number of degenerative conditions which may be seen at school, the most common of which is Duchenne muscular dystrophy.

Duchenne muscular dystrophy

Duchenne muscular dystrophy is a progressive disorder of the skeletal muscles that becomes evident in early childhood. It appears to affect mainly boys. The cause is a genetic defect, which results in changes to muscle fibres thereby reducing strength and flexibility of muscles.

Presenting features

As it is a progressive condition features seen will be dependent on the current stage of development. During later years at school the student may require home tuition. Students with Duchenne muscular dystrophy will experience the following:

Physical symptoms

- weakness in the proximal muscles, starting with hips and then the shoulders;
- frequent falls;
- standing up by walking hands up his leg;
- a waddling/slow gait;
- enlarged calf muscles;
- difficulty climbing stairs;
- decreasing endurance and physical tolerance;
- decreased range of joint movement and flexion contractures at hips, knees and elbows;
- inability to keep up with peers;
- reluctance/inability to run;
- increased weight due to lack of muscle use;
- decreased mobility leading to wheelchair dependence prior to entering secondary school;
- weakness in respiratory muscles;
- laboured speech due to poor breath control.

Social/emotional effects

- low self-esteem and loss of confidence;
- depression;
- loss of motivation;
- increased dependency on others;

Occupational Therapy Approaches for Secondary Special Needs © Whurr Publishers Ltd 2002

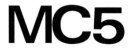
- adjustment to changing role within family and with peer group;
- heightened behavioural problems;
- fear of helplessness and dying;
- difficulty relating to peer group.

Treatment

There is currently no cure for Duchenne muscular dystrophy The student will require different types of intervention at different stages of the condition:

- physiotherapy;
- provision of standing frame for use in school;
- occupational therapy;
- provision of suitable aids and equipment for daily living;
- orthotics – callipers, spinal jacket, ankle/foot orthosis;
- provision of a wheelchair from wheelchair services (via local occupational therapist or physiotherapy departments);
- orthopaedic surgery;
- counselling/emotional support;
- dietician/nutritional advice;
- medication.

Prognosis

Duchenne muscular dystrophy is a progressive disorder; life expectancy is shortened and respiratory failure usually occurs before the person reaches their early twenties.

Further information

Muscular Dystrophy Campaign
7-11 Prescott Place
London SW4 6BS
tel: 020 7720 8055
Email: info@muscular-dystrophy.org
Website: www.muscular-dystrophy.org

Fact sheets are available on the various types and individual conditions of dystrophy.

Regional Officers are employed by the Muscular Dystrophy Campaign to oversee regional activities. Family Care Officers are available to support families and may, circumstances permitting, be available to come into school and talk to staff and year groups.

Further information (continued)

Duchene Family Support Group
37a Highbury New Park
Islington
London N5 2EN
Tel: 0207 7210 8055

Information on aids and communication:

ACE (Aiding Communication in Education)
Centre Advisory Trust
92 Windmill Road
Headington
Oxford OX3 7DR
Tel: 01865 759800
Email: info@ace-centre.org.uk
www.ace-centre.org.uk

ACE Centre Advisory Trust - North
1 Broadbent Road
Watersheddings
Oldham
OL1 4HU
Tel: 0161 6271358
Email: ace-north@ace-north.org
www.ace-centre.org.uk

CALL Centre
University of Edinburgh
Patterson's Land
Hollyrood Road
Edinburgh
EH8 8AQ
Tel: 0131 6516236
Email: call.centre@ed.ac.uk
www.callcentrescotland.org.uk

Refer to information communication technology checklist and resources, Appendix **A3**.

Other degenerative conditions which may be seen in school include:

Spinal muscular atrophy

Spinal muscular atrophy (SMA) is a neuromuscular condition caused by muscle weakness. There are several types of SMA defined by age of onset and severity. For example:

1 *Intermediate - (Type II)*

   ● onset between three months and two years;

   ● may need supportive seating and not be able to stand without an aid;

   ● survival into adulthood possible.

2 *Mild - (Type III) also known as Kugelberg-Nelander disease*

   ● onset usually around two years;

   ● able to walk;

   ● normal lifespan.

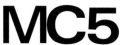

Further information

Consult school doctor or school nurse.

Support is provided by:

The Jennifer Trust for Spinal Muscular Atrophy
Elta House
Birmingham Road
Stratford upon Avon CV37 0AG
Tel: 01789 267520
Email: jennifer@jtsma.org.uk

Becker muscular dystrophy

Becker muscular dystrophy is less severe than Duchenne muscular dystrophy (see above) and is characterized by progressively poor shoulder and pelvic girdle strength. Symptoms begin very mildly in childhood and include cramps during exercise. Later in teen years muscle weakness becomes more evident causing difficulty in rapid walking, running and climbing stairs.

Further information is available from school doctor or school nurse.

Emery-Dreiffus muscular dystrophy

Emery-Dreiffus muscular dystrophy is a muscle-wasting disease characterized by early onset in childhood or adolescence. Muscle contractures develop early before there is any marked muscle weakness. The heart may become affected, necessitating a pacemaker to be fitted. Initial muscle weakness will be evident in the shoulders and upper arms leading to difficulty raising the arms above the head and lifting heavy objects.

Further information

Consult school doctor or school nurse.

Muscular Dystrophy Campaign
7-11 Prescott Place
London SW4 6BS
Tel. 020 7720 8055
Email: info@muscular-dystrophy.org
www.muscular-dystrophy.org

Further reading

Emery AEH (2000) Muscular Dystrophy: The Facts. Oxford: Oxford University Press. (Available from the Muscular Dystrophy Campaign.)
Muscular Dystrophy Campaign (2001) Children with Muscular Dystrophy in Mainstream Schools. (Living fact sheet). London: Muscular Dystrophy Campaign
Reed CL (2001) Quick Reference to Occupational Therapy, 2nd edn. Baltimore, MD: Aspen Publishers.

MC5

Table 2.5 Dystrophies and degenerative conditions

It is essential that

1 A risk assessment is carried out prior to the student entering school and repeated in accordance with the school or county manual handling policy

2 Staff receive regular training in manual handling in accordance with the manual handling policy

3 Staff liaise with the physiotherapist/occupational therapist since damage can occur through inappropriate activities

Students diagnosed with dystrophies/degenerative conditions will present with varying areas of need depending on the severity and stage of their condition. The presenting features below are an extensive list and may not all be relevant.

Management should be targeted for the individual student. It may be necessary to seek advice from your SENCO in order to implement some of these approaches.

Possible Presenting Features	Management Approaches	Further Advice via SENCO
Health – depending on type and severity of condition		
■ Increased weight due to lack of muscle use and exercise	■ Undertake risk assessment Heighten awareness of peers and staff Implications for manual handling, use of a hoist may be necessary Discuss the need to monitor dietary intake with students and parents	■ Refer to school manual handling policy ■ Seek advice from school nurse, doctor, dietician ■ Seek advice from occupational therapist, physiotherapist
■ Spinal deformities, e.g. lordosis/scoliosis	■ Ensure correct seating is available Discuss use of spinal jacket with physiotherapist Ensure physiotherapy programme is timetabled	
■ Possible loss of range of movement in joints/flexion contractures leading to pain when joints are moved	■ Regular physiotherapy programme as directed by the physiotherapist Regular supported standing in frame as directed by physiotherapist	
■ Respiratory muscles often become progressively weaker necessitating time off school due to chest infections	■ Ensure 'missed work' is provided on return to school	
ineffective breath control for speech	Provide means for student to attract attention in class, e.g. buzzer, flashing light Allow extra time for student to speak, particularly during group discussion	

Possible Presenting Features	Management Approaches	Further Advice via SENCO
Health (continued)		
■ Degenerate nature of condition necessitating time out of school for, e.g. hospital appointments, surgery, illness	■ Discuss strategies with parents and students and ensure missed work is passed on to student	
■ 'Off days – although in school, feeling unwell and unable to concentrate	■ Heighten staff and peers' awareness Ensure coping strategies in place, e.g. time out Consider home tuition	
Physical		
■ Mobility reduced stamina, quality of walking and increased possibility of falls	■ Check all equipment available in school, e.g. wheelchair Adult support around school	■ Seek advice from occupational therapist, physiotherapist
reduced mobility eventually leading to wheelchair dependence	■ Check fire exits When planning timetable consider close proximity of classroom and minimize use of stairs Discuss use of wheelchair for transit between lessons Adult support around school Consider student becoming first person in and out of classroom to minimize risk of accidents Limit the amount of walking/mobility around the classroom/laboratory	■ Seek advice from health and safety representative and teacher advisor Discuss with person responsible for timetable planning Seek advice from physiotherapist, wheelchair service
participating in PE/games	■ Discuss with student and physiotherapist PE/games options which are appropriate and attainable to ensure self-esteem is maintained	■ Seek advice from physiotherapist
participating in swimming	■ Do not take swimming without professional advice	■ Seek advice from physiotherapist
reduced endurance and physical tolerance for self-propelling of wheelchair	■ When planning timetables consider close proximity of classroom and accessibility to lifts Adult support around school Provision of an alternative wheelchair in liaison with wheelchair services	■ Discuss with person responsible for timetable planning ■ Contact wheelchair service or occupational therapist regarding provision of wheelchair

Occupational Therapy Approaches for Secondary Special Needs © Whurr Publishers Ltd 2002

MC5 DC (continued)

Table 2.5 Dystrophies and degenerative conditions

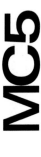

Possible Presenting Features	Management Approaches	Further Advice via SENCO
Physical (continued)		
■ Fine motor gradual reduction in muscle strength and dexterity leading to lack of accuracy when handling instruments/	■ Check student is in optimum position for function, e.g. elbows supported Trial alternative instruments/tools and check appropriate equipment is available Consider buddy/adult support	■ Refer to Occupational Therapy sheet (**OT1**) ■ Seek advice from physiotherapist, occupational therapist or advisory teacher
sustaining handwriting	■ Use a combination of recording methods, e.g. own handwriting, amanuensis, laptop, ICT, part-prepared worksheet Reduce amount of handwriting required	■ Seek advice from ICT advisor Refer to Appendices (**A1** and **A3**)
accessing ICT equipment	■ Investigate alternative ICT equipment, e.g. alternative mouse, reduced sized keyboard, wrist support, touchpad, voice-activated software	■ Seek advice from ICT advisor
Self-care	**Privacy is paramount – discuss with student and parents**	
■ Toileting – access and transfers	■ Undertake risk assessment Ensure adequate space for wheelchair, student and helper Consider rails, hoists, changing table, toilet seat	⎫ ⎪ Seek advice from occupational therapist, physiotherapist, advisory teacher Refer to school manual handling policy
■ Showering – access and transfers	■ Undertake risk assessment Ensure adequate space for wheelchair, student and helper Consider need for supportive equipment, e.g. shower chair, shower bed	⎪
■ Dressing – inability to be totally independent	■ Provide adult support Ensure suitable equipment is available, e.g. hoist, changing table Discuss need for adaptive clothing with parents	⎭

Occupational Therapy Approaches for Secondary Special Needs © Whurr Publishers Ltd 2002

MC5 DC (continued)

Possible Presenting Features	Management Approaches	Further Advice via SENCO

Self-care (continued)

■ Mealtimes
mobility and adequate space around dining hall

obtaining meal from serving hatch
use of cup/cutlery

■ Ensure clear pathways to allow for wheelchair manoeuvrability
Position student at end of table with friends
Assist with opening lunchbox, etc.
Meal collected on wheelchair tray or by friend or adult
Provision of appropriate cutlery/cup
Provide adult support to feed

■ Transferring from wheelchair to chair/toilet/changing bed

■ Undertake risk assessment
Discuss management approach with parents
If student is able to stand independently, practise appropriate transfers after consultation with physiotherapist/occupational therapist
If student is unable to stand, use appropriate hoist – ensure adequate training is given

■ Refer to school manual handling policy and seek advice from pysiotherapist, occupational therapist, advisory teacher

---

Social, emotional and psychological

■ Poor self-concept and low self-esteem, feeling of being different

■ Provide frequent opportunities for student to experience success
Increase staff awareness
Choose peers carefully when planning group work
Provide pastoral support

■ Frustration due to diminished ability

■ Set attainable goals and adapt activity to enhance success
Consider buddy working – choose buddy carefully
Provide pastoral support

■ Depression due to gradual loss of function

■ Discuss concerns with parents
Seek professional support for student
Seek support for teacher from other professionals
Provide opportunities for student to express feelings and emotions

Refer to social interaction skill sheet (F13)

Seek advice from educational psychologist, doctor, child and adolescent mental health service, occupational therapist, physiotherapist, muscular dystrophy field worker

Occupational Therapy Approaches for Secondary Special Needs © Whurr Publishers Ltd 2002

MC5 DC (continued)

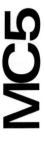

MC5

Table 2.5 Dystrophies and degenerative conditions

Possible Presenting Features	Management Approaches	Further Advice via SENCO
Social, emotional and psychological (continued)		
■ Lack of motivation	■ Ensure lesson/activity is perceived by student to be relevant, interesting and interactive.	Seek advice from educational psychologist, doctor, muscular dystrophy field worker, child and adolescent mental health service, occupational therapist, physiotherapist
■ Student will make greater demands on adult or peers for assistance/attention as condition progresses	■ Make appropriate assessment of need and provide support accordingly Increased awareness by peers and staff of the condition	
■ Heightened behavioural problems	■ Implement behaviour management programme following discussion with psychologist	
■ Fear of helplessness	■ Discuss with parents Provide supportive, non-threatening environment and allow discussion of issues as student raises them	

Juvenile idiopathic arthritis

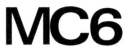

Definition

Juvenile idiopathic arthritis is a chronic condition characterized by inflammation and swelling of one or more joints for at least three months in a child under the age of 16 years. It can start at any age from birth to adolescence but peak age of onset is six years.

Cause

The exact cause has yet to be identified.

What are the main forms of juvenile idiopathic arthritis?

There are three main forms. The condition is characterized by periods of 'flare-ups' followed by periods of remission. Since the condition can become progressive the student's functional abilities will decrease and may result in wheelchair use before leaving school.

Pauciarticular

This is the commonest type of juvenile idiopathic arthritis, accounting for approximately 50% of cases, where up to four joints, e.g. knee, ankle, elbow and hip are affected. The involvement of joints is often asymmetrical and can include inflammation. Sometimes there is damage to the eye, which affects vision.

Polyarticular

This type accounts for almost 20% of cases and affects five or more joints, e.g. hands, wrist, feet, ankle and knee, and sometimes the cervical spine. The involvement of joints is symmetrical and involves pain, swelling and stiffness, plus other symptoms such as weight loss, low grade fever and general malaise.

Systemic (Still's disease)

This type accounts for about 10% of cases and starts with systemic symptoms, e.g. fever, lethargy, enlarged glands. It affects multiple joints and other organ systems including the spleen, liver and lymph nodes.

Presenting features

Students with juvenile idiopathic arthritis may have some of the following features in varying degrees of severity.

1 Physical factors

● joints – painful, inflamed, swollen;
● morning stiffness;

- reduced movement in affected joints, tightness or flexion contractures of affected joints;
- restricted movements giving an appearance of a stiff/stilted gait;
- poor posture;
- joint instability with possibility of subluxation or dislocation;
- muscle wastage around affected joints;
- muscle spasm particularly in hips and knees;

- reduced balance and poor saving reactions;
- weight loss/gain;
- low grade fever;
- general malaise;
- may need wheelchair if joints in lower limb become inflamed.

2 Social/emotional factors

- loss of self-esteem and self-confidence;
- feelings of being different;
- irritable and listless;
- depression;
- fatigue and low endurance;
- dependency on others.

Treatment

There is no cure for juvenile idiopathic arthritis, however the student may be offered different types of intervention including:

- medication;
- joint protection advice;
- pain management programme;
- splinting;
- physiotherapy/hydrotherapy;
- occupational therapy;
- provision of suitable aids and equipment for daily living;
- surgery – potential joint replacement;
- counselling.

Prognosis

Approximately 50–75% of students recover completely within one to two years from the onset of juvenile idiopathic arthritis. About 15% of those with the polyarticular type have permanent disabilities.

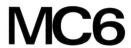
Further information

Arthritis Research Campaign
PO Box 177
Chesterfield
Derbyshire S41 7BR
Tel: 01246 558033
Fax: 01246 558007
Email: info@arc.org.uk
www.arthritiscare.org.uk

Young Arthritis Care
18 Stevenson Way
London NW1 2HD
Tel: 020 7380 6500
Help line: 0808 8000 4050
Email: info@arc.org.uk
www.arthritiscare.org.uk

**Children's Chronic Arthritis
Association (CCAA)**
47 Battenhall Avenue
Worcester WR5 2HN
Tel: 01905 745595

Further reading

Arthritis Care et al (1997) Children Have Arthritis Too (CHAT) - Juvenile Chronic Arthritis. London: Arthritis Care.

Arthritis Care (2001) Chat2Parents – Arthritis in Teenagers. London: Arthritis Care.

Arthritis Research Campaign (1993) When a Young Person Has Arthritis. Chesterfield: Arthritis Research Campaign. (Written for teachers.)

Arthritis Research Campaign (2000) Arthritis in Teenagers. Chesterfield: Arthritis Research Campaign.

Reed,CL (2001) Quick Reference to Occupational Therapy, 2nd edn. Baltimore, MD: Aspen Publishers.

MC6 Joint protection for juvenile idiopathic arthritis

Students with juvenile idiopathic arthritis should learn how to conserve energy and relieve strain placed on an individual joint whilst maintaining the correct balance between activity and rest.

What is joint protection?

- Enabling the student to realize the extent to which they can use their joints.
- Avoiding deformity by using joints correctly.
- Learning to use joints in a way that causes minimal strain.
- Maintaining and improving function rather than restricting it.

When to use joint protection?

It is a way of life and should be used during all activity to prevent overstrain on the joint.

Why use joint protection?

Students may be in pain because they:

- carried out the same movement for too long;
- did not have a break during the activity;
- did work which was too heavy for them.

Principles of joint protection

1   Energy conservation

- beware of fatigue: stop before it occurs;
- alternate heavy and light tasks;
- plan periods of activity followed by periods of rest;
- take regular breaks;
- do not stand if sitting is possible;
- avoid repetitive unnecessary activities;
- seek ways to reduce effort needed to complete task.

2   Relieve strain placed on joints

- distribute load over two or more joints e.g. use both hands;
- use larger, stronger joints and biggest muscles to lift and carry;
- use shoulders instead of hands;
- use hands instead of fingers;

Occupational Therapy Approaches for Secondary Special Needs © Whurr Publishers Ltd 2002

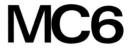

- avoid propping hands under chin when working;
- avoid carrying too much weight – use backpack/bag with diagonal strap;
- avoid static positions, e.g. standing/sitting for long periods of time;
- avoid tight grasp or prolonged grips – use enlarged/lever type handles;
- avoid keeping joints in one position for long periods of time, e.g. holding a pencil.

3   Support joints

- wear splints if supplied;
- use correct techniques when sitting – legs and back should be supported.

REMEMBER

Too much activity results in:

- pain and fatigue;
- overstrain on joints;
- increased inflammation of joints;
- faulty joint positions.

Too much rest results in:

- poor strength;
- faulty joint positions;
- decreased mobility;

MC6

Table 2.6 Juvenile idiopathic arthritis

It is essential that
1 A risk assessment is carried out prior to the student entering school and repeated in accordance with the school or county manual handling policy
2 Staff receive regular training in manual handling in accordance with the manual handling policy
3 Staff liaise with the physiotherapist/occupational therapist since damage can occur through inappropriate activities

Students diagnosed with juvenile idiopathic arthritis will present with varying areas of need depending on the severity and stage of their condition. The presenting features below are an extensive list and may not all be relevant.

Management should be targeted for the individual student. It maybe necessary to seek advice from your SENCO in order to implement some of these approaches.

Possible Presenting Features	Management Approaches	Further Advice via SENCO
Health		
■ Inflammation and swelling of joints leading to painful and reduced range of movement	■ Ensure splints are worn if provided Encourage student to self-monitor energy levels in relation to task and provide appropriate help Follow joint protection procedures (in this section p. 88)	■ Seek advice from occupational therapist, physiotherapist
■ Flexion contractures of joints causing restricted movement	■ Ensure supportive seating is available	■ Refer to Equipment resources (**ER**) Occupational Therapy sheet (**OT1**) Seek advice from occupational therapist, physiotherapist
■ Morning stiffness	■ Heighten staff awareness of additional difficulties in early morning lessons	
■ Risk of joint deformities	■ Analyse physical requirements of task to ensure excessive stress is not put on joints Follow joint protection procedures (in this section p. 88) Ensure splints are worn if provided	■ Seek advice from occupational therapist, physiotherapist
■ Problems sustaining static postures or performing repetitive movements due to muscle spasm in wrist and knee joints	■ Use an alternative functional posture, e.g. perching stool Provide regular opportunities to change position and activity, e.g. every 20–30 minutes Provide buddy/adult support Ensure hand splint is worn if provided	■ Refer to Equipment resources (**ER**)

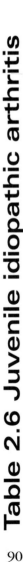

Possible Presenting Features	Management Approaches	Further Advice via SENCO
Health (continued)		
■ Fluctuating nature of condition necessitating time out of school, e.g. hospital appointments, surgery, illness	■ Heighten staff awareness ■ Discuss strategies with parents and students to ensure missed work is passed on to student	■ Seek advice from school nurse/doctor
■ 'Off' days – although in school, feeling unwell and unable to concentrate	■ Heighten staff and peers awareness ■ Ensure coping strategies in place, e.g. time out ■ Provide pastoral support	
Physical gross motor skills		
■ Mobility reduced mobility sometimes resulting in the use of wheelchair or crutches	■ When planning timetable consider proximity of classrooms and minimize use of stairs Consider student being first in/out of classroom to minimize risk of further damage to joints/pain Consider adult support to carry bag or use a backpack Provide locker to reduce need for carrying of equipment	■ Discuss with person responsible for timetable planning
lack of stamina and poor quality of walking	■ When planning timetable consider close proximity of classrooms and minimize use of stairs Limit amount of time walking around classroom/laboratory	■ Discuss with person responsible for timetable planning
difficulty participating in PE/games **Generally, contact sports should be avoided**	■ Discuss with student and physiotherapist PE/games options which are appropriate and attainable within limitations of condition	■ Seek advice from physiotherapist
■ Poor posture affecting functional performance in sitting/standing	■ Ensure supportive seating is available, e.g. perching stool	■ Refer to Equipment resources (**ER**)

Possible Presenting Features	Management Approaches	Further Advice via SENCO
Physical (continued)		
■ Access into buildings including classrooms, toilets, shower, library, canteen	■ Check heights/number of steps/stairs, consider rails/ramps, check door positions/handles and alter if necessary Consider need/viability of through floor lift/stair lift	■ Seek advice from occupational therapist, physiotherapist, advisory teacher, county surveyor
around external school facilities	■ Consider need for rails/ramps or alternative route around site	■ Seek advice from occupational therapist, physiotherapist, advisory teacher
■ School trips/field trips – access, mobility, transport	■ Pre-check access and facilities, e.g. dining area, toilet, parking area Ensure appropriate equipment is available Extra support may be needed	■ Refer to school trips policy
Physical fine motor dexterity		**Refer to fine manual dexterity skill sheet (F2)**
■ Reduced manual dexterity leading to lack of accuracy when handling equipment	■ Ensure splints are worn if provided Check student is in optimum position for function, e.g. forearms and feet supported Trial alternative equipment, instruments, tools Check appropriate equipment is available Follow joint protection procedures (in this section, p. 88) Consider 'buddy'/adult support	■ Seek advice from occupational therapist, physiotherapist, advisory teacher ■ Refer to Equipment resources (**ER**)
■ Sustaining handwriting	■ Use a combination of recording methods e.g. own handwriting, amanuensis, laptop, ICT, part-prepared worksheets Implement energy conservation/pacing strategies (in this section p. 88) Reduce amount of handwriting required	■ Seek advice from ICT advisor ■ Refer to Appendices (**A1** and **A3**)
■ Accessing ICT equipment	■ Investigate use of alternatives e.g. key guard, touch pad, mouse, voice activated software	■ Seek advice from ICT advisor
■ Performing hand and wrist activities, e.g. unscrewing jars, using keys, holding pencil	■ Use adapted equipment Implement joint protection procedures (in this section p. 88)	■ Refer to Equipment resources (**ER**)

Occupational Therapy Approaches for Secondary Special Needs © Whurr Publishers Ltd 2002

MC6 JIA (continued)

Possible Presenting Features	Management Approaches	Further Advice via SENCO
Self-care	**Privacy is paramount. Discuss with student and parents**	
■ Access to toilet and carrying out toileting procedures	■ Ensure adequate space Provide rails and lever taps	Seek advice from occupational therapist, physiotherapist, advisory teacher
■ Showering	■ Ensure shower is available with level access, rail, lever taps and seat	
■ Slow at dressing/managing clothing, fastenings	■ Ensure clothing/fastenings are adapted e.g. skirts/trousers with elasticated waists, velcro fastenings, elastic laces Use dressing aids if appropriate Allow extra time Provide adult help	■ Seek advice from occupational therapist
■ Mealtimes		
mobility and adequate space around dining hall	■ Ensure clear pathways to allow for manoeuvrability	
obtaining meal from serving area and handling money	■ Share tray with friend. Ask friend/dinner lady to help with money	
awkward use of cutlery	■ Provision of appropriate equipment	■ Seek advice from occupational therapist
Social, emotional and psychological		**Refer to social interaction skill sheet (F13)**
■ Poor self-concept, low self-esteem, feelings of being different	■ Provide frequent opportunities for student to experience success Increase staff awareness to the condition Choose peers carefully when planning group work Provide pastoral support	Seek advice from child and adolescent mental health service occupational therapist, school nurse, physiotherapist
■ Frustrated due to diminished ability or pain in affected joints	■ Set attainable goals and adapt activity Consider buddy working – choose buddy carefully Provide pastoral support	

Table 2.6 Juvenile idiopathic arthritis

Possible Presenting Features	Management Approaches	Further Advice via SENCO
Social, emotional and psychological (continued)		
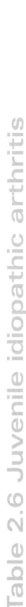 Depressed, irritable, moody, listless due to impaired functional ability and/or pain	■ Discuss concerns with parents Seek professional support for student Provide opportunities to express feelings and emotions Frequent teacher feedback and redirection	Seek advice from child and adolescent mental health service occupational therapist, school nurse, physiotherapist
■ Variable/intense pain in joints leading to withdrawal, hostility and reluctance to participate	■ Implementation of pain management programme	
■ Providing/varying appropriate level of assistance in relation to student's day-to-day functional abilities	■ Discuss with student and parents Encourage student to be proactive and request/accept help as needed	

Chapter 3
Curriculum areas

Introduction

The expectations for students transferring from primary to secondary school are enormous. Students generally leave a small, close-knit community to become members of a much larger community where they are encouraged to work towards becoming independent and planning their own programmes of study. For many students this creates a challenge, but for those with special needs the task is even harder, especially as different teachers will employ a variety of teaching styles.

It is therefore important for subject teachers to be aware that a student's delayed development of foundation skills will have an impact on his or her performance in class. When learning new skills, students need to build on previous achievements. Foundation skills are the building blocks enabling students to move from one skill base to the next.

Many core foundation skills are cross-curricular, necessitating the information to be repeated from one subject to another. Each subject has its own curriculum requirements and these have also been analysed in the subject tables (see Tables 3.1–3.11).

When using these tables, it should be recognized that some of the practical strategies will need preparation time prior to the student attending the lesson. The special educational needs co-ordinator (SENCO) will be able to identify who should implement approaches and strategies in a particular subject area. Some strategies may also be applicable to students who have not been identified with a particular medical condition, but display similar behaviour.

An individual student profile sheet is included in the Appendices (**A6**) for easy transfer of specific practical approaches and strategies for a particular student.

Each subject area has been presented as a complete 'package', so that information can be quickly and effectively disseminated to relevant staff, possibly by highlighting the appropriate sections. The SENCO and learning support staff will have set targets for a student's individual education plan, so they will be aware of the personnel involved in achieving the desirable outcomes. When considering the further advice column, it is advisable that the SENCO is always consulted prior to any outside agency becoming involved with the student.

Table 3.1 English

Possible Classroom Problem	Possible Practical Approach	Further Advice via SENCO
Gross motor co-ordination	**It may be necessary to seek advice from your SENCO in order to implement some of these approaches**	**Refer to gross motor co-ordination skill sheet (F1)**
■ Ability to maintain functional writing posture	■ Check sitting posture – chair/table size and height Consider angled surface, e.g. clipboard, lever arch file Provide rise and fall table with tilting surface	■ Refer to Occupational Therapy sheet (**OT1**), Equipment resources (**ER**) ■ Refer to Equipment resources (**ER**)
■ Reduced stamina for extended periods of writing Reduced quantity of written work, which will include completion of homework	■ Alternative recording methods, e.g. appropriate ICT, voice-activated computer software, dictaphone, part-prepared worksheets with spacing to reduce the amount of copying Consider adult support as an amanuensis Encourage editing of work Use bullet points rather than full sentence construction, e.g. use 'writing frames' Give realistic targets – set attainable goals Consider extending time to complete task Consider extra time allowance in exams and fatigue breaks Allow student to re-establish posture by standing, stretching, etc. at agreed time intervals, i.e. every 15 minutes Record homework using dictaphone/tape recorder for transcribing later Attend homework club (arranged by SENCO) if student is not too tired	■ Seek advice from ICT advisor and refer to Appendices (**A1** and **A3**) ■ Refer to Further reading ■ Seek advice from educational psychologist
■ Mobility around the classroom	■ Identify safe route by avoiding bags, feet, etc. Keep pathways clear Review position in class – consider sitting at end of row/table or near aisle	

Possible Classroom Problem	Possible Practical Approach	Further Advice via SENCO
Fine motor dexterity	**It may be necessary to seek advice from your SENCO in order to implement some of these approaches**	**Refer to fine motor dexterity skill sheet (F2)**
■ Neatness of handwriting and presentation of work	■ Check sitting posture – chair/table size and height Consider working on an angled surface, e.g. clipboard, lever-arch file	■ Refer to Occupational Therapy sheet (**OT1**) and Equipment resources (**ER**)
Fluency and speed of handwriting	Encourage cursive script to increase flow/fluency Use lined paper to help with letter placement Consider alternative pencil grasps and trial different writing tools Consider amanuensis Accept that quantity of written work will be reduced Encourage pressure awareness–consider paper textures	■ Refer to Occupational Therapy sheet (**OT1**) and Equipment resources (**ER**) ■ Refer to Occupational Therapy sheet (**OT1**) ■ Seek advice from ICT advisor
	Consider alternative recording methods, e.g. appropriate ICT, voice-activated computer software, dictaphone, part-prepared worksheets with spaces for student to fill in Consider extra time allowance or adult support as a scribe in exam situations	■ Seek advice from educational pyschologist
■ Submitting incomplete homework	Record homework on dictaphone for transcribing later Provide part-prepared notes and worksheets Consider student's difficulties when setting work	
■ Using information communications technology (ICT) equipment due to reduced skills for keyboard and mouse	■ Consider support to set up and carry equipment Provide sufficient forearm support – use appropriate size of table, wrist rest/support Colour code keyboard Teach touch-typing Try alternative mouse devices Use 'dampening' facility to reduce repetition when key is depressed for too long Use key guard to improve accuracy	■ Refer to Equipment resources (**ER**) ■ Seek advice from ICT advisor and refer to Appendix (**A3**) ■ Refer to Equipment resources (**ER**)
■ Using instruments, e.g. rulers, scissors	■ Trial alternative equipment Consider buddy working/adult support	■ Refer to Equipment resources (**ER**)

Table 3.1 English

Possible Classroom Problem	Possible Practical Approach	Further Advice via SENCO
Organizational skills	**It may be necessary to seek advice from your SENCO in order to implement some of these approaches**	**Refer to organizational skill sheet (F3)**
■ Preparation for school day and subject	■ Additional training to use school organizer Use a daily timetable and different coloured dots for each subject Colour code books to correspond with subjects, e.g. Maths blue, English red (use coloured plastic exercise book covers) List books/items needed for each subject. Use coloured zipped plastic wallets	■ Refer to Occupational Therapy sheet (**OT7**)
■ Presentation and layout of written work	■ Cue sheet showing sample layout – concrete example, visual plan Use part-prepared sheets Use pre-prepared format with spaces for beginning, middle and end points Jot down essential points to be included, order and number them before writing in full format, crossing off from jotting sheet Use 'writing frames' Use a different colour for beginning, middle and end points in the rough draft Fold paper or draw extra lines to reinforce awareness of columns, e.g. indentations for poems Use lined/squared paper and pre-ruled margins	■ Refer to Further reading
■ Using indexes/dictionaries	■ Provide an alphabet strip – stick on ruler or keep in pencil case Colour code alphabet strip, e.g. abc-red, def-blue, ghi-green Use dictionaries with tabs and clear, bold print on top of each page	
■ Organizing work area/desk	■ Only essential items in work area – use a checklist Adult/peer support Consider position in class, e.g. position student so left- and right-handed students are not colliding Encourage student to store work in appropriate folder/pocket file	

Possible Classroom Problem	Possible Practical Approach	Further Advice via SENCO

Organizational Skills (continued)

Possible Classroom Problem	Possible Practical Approach	Further Advice via SENCO
■ Using information communications technology (ICT) equipment	■ Diagrammatic step-by-step guide on how to set up equipment and cue cards for more specific tasks Designated bag to carry ICT equipment in with contents list Use labels to identify discs Ensure student is familiar with software	■ Seek advice from school ICT department
■ Ability to follow verbal instructions	■ Reinforce with written notes Give instructions in small steps and repeat instructions Ask student to repeat instructions to check he or she has heard and understood. If possible withdraw to quiet area and give assistance Provide assistance to ensure homework instructions are understood – use a homework diary	■ Seek advice from speech and language therapist
■ Ability to follow written instructions	■ Break down instructions into small steps Write instructions in point form, underline/highlight key instructions Withdraw to quiet area and give assistance Consider buddy working/adult assistance	
■ Expressive skills, e.g. argument, debate, analysis Critical analysis of literature	■ Give prompts (verbal or written) Ask leading questions. Allow time for student to answer Use mind-mapping techniques	■ Seek advice from educational psychologist, speech and language therapist ■ Refer to Further reading
■ Selecting appropriate information from written text	■ Provide a cue card listing information to look for in text Use highlighters/colour coding systems Provide cues or write words in margin e.g. as prompts Use line tracker, appropriate-sized windows, clear ruler to highlight specific areas	■ Refer to Equipment resources (**ER**)
■ Paraphrasing	■ Reinforce study skills	■ Refer to Further reading

CA1 English (continued)

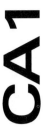

CA1

Table 3.1 English

Possible Classroom Problem	Possible Practical Approach	Further Advice via SENCO
Visual motor integration	**It may be necessary to seek advice from your SENCO in order to implement some of these approaches**	**Refer to visual motor integration skill sheet (F6)**
■ Producing illustrations to enhance work	■ Use alternatives e.g. Clip Art™, computer graphics, pre-drawn work only needing to be labelled, commercially available stencils/templates Allow student to trace illustrations from books Adult support to produce illustrations for student	
■ Neatness and presentation of handwriting	■ Check sitting posture to ensure student is sitting in optimum working position Provide notes and worksheets to reduce the amount of writing Use bullet points rather than full sentence construction Use 'writing frames' Use appropriate lined paper to help with letter placement Use alternative recording methods e.g. appropriate ICT, dictaphone, adult support as a scribe Consider allowing longer time to complete task Consider extra time allowance/adult support as a scribe in exam situations	■ Refer to Occupational Therapy sheet (**OT1**) ■ Refer to Further reading ■ Seek advice from ICT advisor and refer to Appendices (**A1** and **A3**) ■ Seek advice from educational pyschologist
Visual spatial relationships	**It may be necessary to seek advice from your SENCO in order to implement some of these approaches**	**Refer to visual spatial relationships skill sheet (F7)**
■ Writing on the line	■ Use a physical barrier as a prompt to keep on line, e.g. 'Stop/go' paper	■ Refer to Equipment resources (**ER**)
■ Uniformity e.g. of shape, size, spacing and slope of letters	■ Use of squared/lined paper to help sizing and placing Use prompt card for word spacing Encourage self-monitoring by using 'rules for writing tasks'	■ Refer to Occupational Therapy sheet (**OT3**)

Possible Classroom Problem	Possible Practical Approach	Further Advice via SENCO
Visual spatial relationships (continued)		
■ Interpreting and producing a range of layouts/formats, e.g. advertisements, newspapers, letters	■ Pre-prepared templates in various shapes and sizes to help arrange layout before transferring to paper Give concrete example of expected format Use part-prepared layout Use appropriate-sized windows to block out unwanted text	
■ Linear and vertical scanning	■ Reinforce working left to right, top to bottom and use of margin as a reference point Use clear/perspex ruler as a line tracker Produce work on squared paper to help with scanning/placement	■ Refer to Foundation skill sheet (**F5**) and Appendix (**A4**)
■ Drama/plays	■ Allow extra time to orientate around stage area Identify concrete points of reference on the stage area, e.g. left/right exit arrows in red/green Give cue cards stating stage direction specific to student's movements on the stage Reinforce understanding of non-verbal language, e.g. personal space Use buddy support/partner working	
Visual figure ground discrimination	**It may be necessary to seek advice from your SENCO in order to implement some of these approaches**	**Refer to visual figure ground skill sheet (F9)**
■ Preparation for lesson in general	■ Ensure personal timetable is not too cluttered and that student can read it Limit amount of information on a page/board Limit amount of copying from board Reduce clutter on table or board Colour or highlight key information on page or board	■ Refer to Foundation skill sheet (**F5**), Appendix (**A4**)
■ Selecting information from dictionary/indexes/multiple choice sheet	■ Use line trackers, windows paper to highlight specific area or exclude unwanted text Increase size of print/spacing when preparing multiple choice sheets	■ Refer to Equipment resources (**ER**)

Occupational Therapy Approaches for Secondary Special Needs © Whurr Publishers Ltd 2002

Table 3.1 English

Possible Classroom Problem	Possible Practical Approach	Further Advice via SENCO
Visual figure ground discrimination (continued)		
■ Finding place e.g. in text e.g. plays, poems	■ Try using coloured overlays Use an appropriate-sized window to reduce visual information or a line tracker to help scanning	■ Refer to Foundation skill sheet (**F5**) Seek advice from advisory teacher
■ Proof reading and editing	■ Reinforce scanning left to right, top to bottom Consider using different formats (e.g. fonts, type face, blocking, bullet points, bold) to highlight key points Underline or highlight each new section or new character Highlight specific part to be read in play Use of line tracker to help scanning	■ Refer to Equipment resources (**ER**)
■ Paraphrasing	■ Encourage student to read aloud to notice mistakes – may need to withdraw to a quiet area Use hand-held spellchecker when proof-reading for spelling Use pre-prepared cue card listing words that are consistently difficult for student to spell Use a line tracker	■ Refer to Equipment resources (**ER**) ■ Refer to Equipment resources (**ER**)

Occupational Therapy Approaches for Secondary Special Needs © Whurr Publishers Ltd 2002

Possible Classroom Problem	Possible Practical Approach	Further Advice via SENCO
Visual form constancy	**It may be necessary to seek advice from your SENCO in order to implement some of these approaches**	**Refer to visual form constancy skill sheet (F8)**
■ Handwriting – difficulty developing fast, fluent script	■ Heighten staff awareness to student's difficulty Use alternative methods of recording, e.g. appropriate ICT, adult support as a scribe, part-prepared worksheets	■ Seek advice from ICT advisor and refer to Appendices (**A3** and **A1**)
■ Recognizing the same letter/word when presented in different handwriting styles, type face, font	■ Heighten staff awareness Consider buddy working/adult support Ensure work is presented in a consistent handwriting style, typeface, font where possible	
Visual memory/sequential memory	**It may be necessary to seek advice from your SENCO in order to implement some of these approaches**	**Refer to visual memory/sequential memory skill sheet (F11)**
■ Spelling	■ Use a variety of dictionaries, e.g. ACE dictionaries for phonetic spelling Practise recognition of visual patterns through games, e.g. shape blocks Break down difficult words into patterns thus enabling student to learn through visual sequences Use hand-held spell checker or computer software with in-built spell checker Use alternative computer software, e.g. predictive writer	■ Refer to Equipment resources (**ER**) ■ Refer to Equipment resources (**ER**) ■ Seek advice from ICT advisor
■ Copying information from board	■ Reduce copying from board, e.g. use pre-prepared work sheets or give own copy of board information Check student's position in class relative to board – position near and facing board. Be aware of objects, in line of vision, which may interfere with view Ask teacher to use different colours to differentiate sections of text to be copied Use stickers on board as visual markers Give adequate time for student to record work	■ Refer to Foundation skill sheet (**F5**)

Possible Classroom Problem	Possible Practical Approach	Further Advice via SENCO
Visual memory/sequential memory (continued)		
■ Copying information from book/paper	■ Reduce copying from book, e.g. use pre-prepared worksheets Ask adult to use colours to differentiate sections of text to be copied Explore optimum book/paper position for ease of scanning	■ Refer to Foundation skill sheet (**F5**)
■ Finding work on laptop/wordprocessor	■ Keep a hard copy of all named files Group files under subject/topic headings and use file manager	
■ Making notes	■ Use adult to check through notes Provide word bank of common misspelt words	
Auditory processing and memory	**It may be necessary to seek advice from your SENCO in order to implement some of these approaches**	**Refer auditory processing and memory skill sheet (F12)**
■ Following and remembering verbal instructions	■ Use dictaphone Give clear, concise instructions in small steps Repeat instructions and allow student to verbalize back to check they have heard and understood Reinforce with written notes If possible withdraw student to quiet area and give assistance	■ Seek advice from speech and language therapist
■ Group discussion, e.g. ability to sift, summarize, use salient points, cite evidence	■ Frequent resumé of essential points by group leader Encourage student to record main points of discussion and write down any questions during discussion Ask student leading questions as a prompt Use mind-mapping techniques Allow time for student to answer	■ Seek advice from educational psychologist, speech and language therapist ■ Refer to Further reading

Possible Classroom Problem	Possible Practical Approach	Further Advice via SENCO

Auditory processing and memory (continued)

Possible Classroom Problem	Possible Practical Approach	Further Advice via SENCO
■ Participation in scripted play	■ Give appropriate parts Give separate sheets for each act Encourage student to make own prompt sheet Provide extra time to learn lines and practise cueing Use 'walkie talkie' to cue pupil on stage Use video to reinforce 'flow' of play	
■ Listening e.g. and responding in discussions	■ Give advance warning of forthcoming discussion Check position in class, e.g. sitting in front or facing speaker Use buddy working/adult support Use pre-prepared cue cards	
■ Spelling and phonological processing	■ Break down difficult words into patterns thus enabling student to learn through visual sequences	■ Seek advice from speech and language therapist

Social interaction

Possible Classroom Problem	Possible Practical Approach	Further Advice via SENCO
	It may be necessary to seek advice from your SENCO in order to implement some of these approaches	**Refer to social interaction skill sheet (F13)**
■ Developing communication skills – ability to interpret and evaluate language	■ Refer to social skills training programme, e.g. PSRE syllabus	■ Seek advice from speech and language therapist, educational pyschologist, child and adolescent mental health service
■ Appropriate use of language, e.g. discussion debate	■ Plan and initiate working groups with clear guidelines, e.g. debating rules	
■ Play reading/role play – ability to assume role/react in character; insufficient information to assume character role	■ Use video, mime and role-play to help develop spontaneous responses Discuss role with partner/group members Allow extra time to practise	

Occupational Therapy Approaches for Secondary Special Needs © Whurr Publishers Ltd 2002

Table 3.1 English

106

Possible Classroom Problem	Possible Practical Approach	Further Advice via SENCO
Social interaction (continued)		
■ Awareness of personal space, own and others	■ Social skills training programme Heighten awareness of staff and peers to students difficulty	■ Seek advice from speech and language therapist, educational pyschologist, child and adolescent mental health service
■ Working as part of a group	■ Select group members carefully Allocate an achievable task to student Consider adult facilitation	
■ Ability to pick up appropriate cues, e.g. in play reading, drama, group work	■ Social skills training programme Partner working	
■ Impulsiveness	■ Give student an agreed object to 'fiddle' with Heighten teachers' and peers' awareness Discuss appropriate behaviour management approaches with student and educational pyschologist/behavioural support team	

CA2

Table 3.2 Mathematics

Possible Classroom Problem	Possible Practical Approach	Further Advice via SENCO
Gross motor co-ordination	**It may be necessary to seek advice from your SENCO in order to implement some of these approaches**	**Refer to gross motor co-ordination skill sheet (F1)**
■ Ability to maintain e.g. functional writing posture	■ Check chair/table size and height Consider working on an angled surface, e.g. clipboard, lever-arch file Consider rise and fall table with tilting surface	■ Refer to Occupational Therapy sheet (**OT1**) ■ Refer to Equipment resources (**ER**) ■ Refer to Equipment resources (**ER**)
■ Using large mathematical equipment, e.g. metre sticks, tapes, etc.	■ Consider buddy working/adult support Consider fatigue breaks	
■ Body awareness/organization in practical group work	■ Partner/buddy working Be aware of student's need for extra space Try postural alternatives, e.g. sitting/kneeling/standing	■ Seek advice from physiotherapist, occupational therapist, advisory teachers
■ Mobility around classroom and collection of necessary equipment	■ Consider the environment, e.g. reduce the clutter Review sitting position in class – consider sitting at the end of table/row or near an aisle Reduce need to move around class, e.g. provide individual set of equipment Consider buddy working/adult support One group collects equipment at a time	

Table 3.2 Mathematics

Possible Classroom Problem	Possible Practical Approach	Further Advice via SENCO
Fine motor dexterity	**It may be necessary to seek advice from your SENCO in order to implement some of these approaches**	**Refer to fine motor dexterity skill sheet (F2)**
■ Neatness of recording and presentation of work	■ Check sitting posture, e.g. chair/table size and height Use appropriate lined/squared paper to help numbers, letters sit on the line Consider working on angled surface, e.g. clipboard, lever-arch file Consider using alternative recording methods, e.g. stamps appropriate ICT, dictaphone, part-prepared worksheets Set attainable goals	■ Refer to Occupational Therapy sheet (**OT1**) ■ Refer to Equipment resources (**ER**) ■ Seek advice from ICT advisor, refer to Appendices (**A1** and **A3**)
■ Using instruments, e.g. ruler, protractor, compass, scissors	■ Trial alternative equipment Provide individual set of adapted equipment Consider adult support/buddy working Consider stabilizing equipment, e.g. use dycem matting	■ Refer to Equipment resources (**ER**) Seek advice from occupational therapist, advisory teacher ■ Refer to Equipment resources (**ER**)
■ Drawing accurate diagrams and graphs	■ Use appropriate ICT, e.g. Clip Art™, computer graphics Use a larger scale for graphs/diagrams Set short, attainable goals Provision of part-prepared worksheets, needing to be labelled Allow student to trace the drawings from text book Use of commercially available stencils/templates Consider adult support	
■ Reduced keyboard and mouse skills affecting ability to use ICT equipment	■ Provide sufficient forearm support – use appropriate sized table, wrist support/rest Consider adult support to set up and help carry equipment Use a key guard to improve accuracy Try alternative mouse devices and keyboards Use 'dampening' facility to reduce repetition when keys are depressed for too long	■ Refer to Occupational Therapy sheet (**OT1**) ■ Refer to Equipment resources (**ER**) ■ Refer to Equipment resources (**ER**) ■ Seek advice from ICT advisor, refer to Appendix (**A3**)
■ Using a calculator due to reduced finger accuracy	■ Trial different calculators	■ Refer to Equipment resources (**ER**)

Occupational Therapy Approaches for Secondary Special Needs © Whurr Publishers Ltd 2002

CA2 Mathematics (continued)

Possible Classroom Problem	Possible Practical Approach	Further advice via SENCO
	It may be necessary to seek advice from your SENCO in order to implement some of these approaches	Refer to organizational skill sheet (F3)
Organizational skills		
■ Presentation and layout of work	■ Provide cue sheet showing sample layout – visual plan Use larger scale for graphs/diagrams Use lined/squared/isometric paper Fold paper or draw extra lines to reinforce awareness of columns Use alternative recording methods e.g. appropriate ICT, use pre-prepared work sheets, adult support to scribe, stencils, number stamps	■ Seek advice from ICT advisor, refer to Appendices (**A1** and **A3**)
■ Performing practical tasks, e.g. using rulers, protractor, compass, scissors	■ Try alternative equipment Have all essential equipment on table before starting task – use cue cards/lists Buddy working/adult support	■ Refer to Equipment resources (**ER**), seek advice from advisory teacher, occupational therapist
■ Organizing work area/desk	■ Only essential items in work area – use a checklist Consider using 'work schedules' Adult or peer support Consider position in class, e.g. place student so left- and right-handed pupils are not colliding Provide student with extra space; student may need their own desk/table	■ Refer to Occupational Therapy sheet (**OT7**) ■ Refer to Appendix (**A5**)
■ Using ICT equipment	■ Provide diagrammatic, step-by-step guide on how to set up equipment and cue cards for more specific tasks Ensure student uses labels to identify discs Ensure student is familiar with software Designated bag to carry equipment in with contents list	■ Seek advice from school ICT department
■ Ability to follow verbal instructions	■ Reinforce with written/pictorial/diagrammatic notes Give instructions in small steps and repeat instructions as required–frequent recapping of instructions Consider adult assistance to ensure homework instructions are understood and written down, e.g. in homework diary	■ Seek advice from speech and language therapist

CA2 Mathematics (continued)

Table 3.2 Mathematics

Possible Classroom Problem	Possible Practical Approach	Further Advice via SENCO
Organizational skills (continued)		
■ Ability to follow written instructions	■ Underline/highlight key parts of instruction Give assistance to ensure that homework instructions are clear and understood	
■ Formulas and equations remembering/sequencing substituting number for letter (e.g. in algebra)	■ Provide cue cards listing formulas/equations Break formulas/equations down and colour code sections.	
■ Difficulty generalizing principles	■ Raise awareness of need to teach individual stages of process as student will not automatically generalize concepts	
Visual motor integration	**It may be necessary to seek advice from your SENCO in order to implement some of these approaches**	**Refer to visual motor integration skill sheet (F6)**
■ Inaccurate manipulative skills due to poor eye-hand co-ordination, e.g. for protractor, ruler, compass	■ Check posture and ensure stability with elbows resting on bench Consider adult support when accuracy is paramount Trial alternative equipment	■ Refer to Occupational Therapy sheet (**OT1**) ■ Refer to Equipment resources (**ER**), seek advice from advisory teacher, occupational therapist
■ Copying 2D shapes and drawing shapes in general	■ Use multi-sensory approaches, teach through use of concrete shape Use alternatives, e.g. stickers, stencils, templates, pre-drawn shapes, computer graphics Allow student to trace drawings from text book	■ Refer to Equipment resources (**ER**)
■ Drawing adjacent/overlapping/interlocking shapes	■ Look and talk about position of shapes and task required Use concrete examples and explain how end product is formed. Use highlighter pen to outline shape	
■ Judging perspective/angles	■ Use a point of reference Have concrete examples Use a protractor	

Occupational Therapy Approaches for Secondary Special Needs © Whurr Publishers Ltd 2002

CA2 Mathematics (continued)

Possible Classroom Problem	Possible Practical Approach	Further Advice via SENCO
Visual spatial relationships	It may be necessary to seek advice from your SENCO in order to implement some of these approaches	**Refer to visual spatial relationships skill sheet (F7)**
■ Using linear and vertical scanning	■ Reinforce working left to right, top to bottom and use of margin, e.g. colour margin red or green, work to margin in book Use clear perspex ruler as a line tracker or for grids use two rulers positioned at 90 degrees to one another Use squared/isometric paper to help scanning/placing	■ Refer to Foundation skill sheet (**F5**), Appendix (**A4**)
■ Interpreting and reproducing symmetry of 2D/3D shapes	■ Provide concrete examples of 2D and 3D shapes for student to manipulate	
■ Making reflection/rotation/enlargements and combinations in 2D	■ Provide concrete examples of 2D object Label parts on previously drawn examples Use isometric paper Photocopy a grid onto an acetate and place over work	
■ Drawing 2D representation of 3D objects	■ Work on squared/isometric paper. Give instructions on how to transfer 3D to 2D Teach 'rules' on how to draw common shapes Draw for student or use stencils, templates Allow student to trace diagrams from text book	
■ Analysing patterns	■ Label significant features on previous examples	
■ Understanding scale – using and interpreting when drawing	■ Use graph paper as visual cue of size representation or use scale ruler	
■ Understanding fractions	■ Provide visual representation/concrete object	
■ Drawing common 2D shapes in different orientation on grids	■ Use appropriate ICT, e.g. computer graphics, Clip Art™ Work on squared/isometric paper Instruct student on how to change orientation of shapes Manipulate templates of shapes into different orientations on grid	

Occupational Therapy Approaches for Secondary Special Needs © Whurr Publishers Ltd 2002

Table 3.2 Mathematics

Possible Classroom Problem	Possible Practical Approach	Further Advice via SENCO
Visual spatial relationships (continued)		
■ Presentation and layout of work	■ Use graph or scaled paper to assist with correct placement Use pre-drawn tables, diagrams, axis for graphs highlighting data using different colours Use line tracker/appropriate-sized window/right angled guide to help placement Discuss layout and provide proforma	■ Refer to Equipment resources (**ER**)
■ Estimating length/depth/height	■ Use concrete examples Use graph paper as a visual cue of size representation Use 'large' measuring equipment	
Visual figure ground discrimination	**It may be necessary to seek advice from your SENCO in order to implement some of these approaches**	**Refer to visual figure ground skill sheet (F9)**
■ Reading information on the page/board	■ Limit amount of information on a page/board Colour code or highlight key information e.g. on page/board Limit amount of copying from board Check student's position in class relative to board – if possible position near and facing board	■ Refer to Foundation skill sheet (**F5**), Appendix (**A4**)
■ Drawing and interpreting graphs, spreadsheet, tables, bar charts, pie charts, shapes, etc.	■ Use pre-drawn graphs, bar/pie charts, highlighting key data Use larger scale Enlarge work sheets Limit the amount of information on each page, e.g. one graph on a page instead of four Encourage student to highlight whilst working Use an appropriate sized window to reduce visual information or a line tracker to help scanning Use appropriate computer software e.g. Clip Art™	

Possible Classroom Problem	Possible Practical Approach	Further Advice via SENCO

Visual figure ground discrimination (continued)

■ Reading and interpreting computer printouts
Using and interpreting data sheets/lists

■ Use larger print to reduce information on a sheet
Use double-spaced print to reduce cluttered appearance
Colour or highlight key information before lesson
Encourage student to highlight whilst working
Use an appropriate-sized window to reduce visual information or a line tracker to help scanning

■ Refer to Equipment resources (**ER**)

■ Multiple-choice questions within the same page

■ Highlight relevant part of question if it corresponds to several options
Increase size of print and spacing, e.g. by enlarging on photocopier or whilst drawing on computer
Use an appropriate-sized window to reduce visual information or a line tracker to help scanning

■ Refer to Equipment resources (**ER**)

■ Using and interpreting scale on maps and drawings

■ Use graph/squared paper to give visual representation of size and scale.

■ Obtaining measurements, e.g. reading scales

■ Consider alternative equipment with clearer markings
Alter position of body to find optimum visual acuity
Ensure good contrast between material and scale

■ Refer to Foundation skill sheet (**F5**)

■ Organization and layout of overlapping drawings

■ Use clear, uncluttered prepared worksheets to limit amount of drawing
Allow student to trace drawings from text book
Use squared/graph paper

Table 3.2 Mathematics

Possible Classroom Problem	Possible Practical Approach	Further Advice via SENCO
Visual form constancy	**It may be necessary to seek advice from your SENCO in order to implement some of these approaches**	**Refer to visual form constancy skill sheet (F8)**
■ Classifying shapes	■ Discuss essential properties of shapes Provide concrete examples to manipulate, e.g. Meccano-type equipment Initially use pictures/items of the same (or as similar as possible) size and colour/design	
■ Recognizing relationship between 2D and 3D shapes, e.g. picture of cube with actual cube	■ Use concrete examples to manipulate, e.g. Meccano-type equipment Label significant features on examples	
■ Investigating common properties of shape	■ Provide list outlining common features to enable student to classify	
■ Making representative 3D models	■ Provide part or completed models	
■ Drawing common 2D shapes in different orientations on grid	■ Use appropriate ICT Software, e.g. Clip Art™, computer graphics Work on squared paper/isometric paper Instruct student on how to change orientation of shape by using concrete examples Use stickers, stencils, templates, pre-drawn shapes Relate properties of drawing to concrete object	■ Refer to Equipment resources (ER)
Visual closure	**It may be necessary to seek advice from your SENCO in order to implement some of these approaches**	**Refer to visual closure skill sheet (F10)**
■ Being able to 'see' complete formulas, equations	■ Use prompt cards	
■ Identifying and locating objects on table when only part of object is visible	■ Maintain clear, organized work surfaces	

Occupational Therapy Approaches for Secondary Special Needs © Whurr Publishers Ltd 2002

Possible Classroom Problem	Possible Practical Approach	Further Advice via SENCO
visual memory/sequential memory	**It may be necessary to seek advice from your SENCO in order to implement some of these approaches**	**Refer to visual memory/sequential memory skill sheet (F11)**
■ Copying from the board	■ Reduce copying from board, e.g. use part-prepared work sheets, give own copy of board information Check students position in class – relative to board, position near and facing board Be aware of objects, in line of vision, which could interfere with student's view Ask teacher to use different colours to differentiate sections of text to be copied Use stickers on board as visual marker Be aware that it will take student longer to copy work and give adequate time for work to be recorded	
■ Copying number and shape patterns	■ Trace pattern with finger before drawing Talk through pattern Give cue card listing equations/pattern Break equations down and colour code sections	
■ Remembering equations, formulas	■ Provide cue card listing equations, formulas pattern Break down equations and colour code sections	
Auditory processing and memory	**It may be necessary to seek advice from your SENCO in order to implement some of these approaches**	**Refer to auditory processing/memory skill sheet (F12)**
■ Following and remembering verbal instructions	■ Use dictaphone Give clear, concise instructions in small steps Repeat instructions and allow student to verbalize back to check that they have heard and understood – frequent recapping of instructions Reinforce with written notes, visual cues If possible withdraw student to quiet area and give assistance	■ Seek advice from speech and language therapist

Table 3.2 Mathematics

Possible Classroom Problem	Possible Practical Approach	Further Advice via SENCO
Auditory processing and memory (continued)		
■ Mental arithmetic problems	■ Reinforce with written notes, visual cues 　Use mnemonics 　Use mind maps/cognitive maps 　Teach how to draw out main factors to solve problem 　e.g. record numbers, record sign(s) involved	■ Refer to Further reading
■ Learning multiplication tables, e.g. 10 × 10	■ Link visual reinforcement with motor task, i.e. look, listen, do 　Provide multiplication tables 　Use finger tables 　Use mind maps/cognitive maps	■ Refer to Further reading
Social interaction	**It may be necessary to seek advice from your SENCO in order to implement some of these approaches**	**Refer to social interaction sheet (F13)**
■ Awareness of personal space (own and others)	■ Heighten teachers' and peers' awareness to student's difficulty 　Social skills training programme/refer to PRSE materials	■ Seek advice from child and adolescent mental health service, educational pychologist
■ Impulsiveness	■ Heighten teachers' and peers' awareness to student's difficulty 　Consider use of 'work schedules' 　Encourage student to pre-plan task	■ Refer to Appendix (**A5**)
■ Working as part of a group	■ Select group members carefully 　Allocate student achievable task 　Consider adult facilitation	

Occupational Therapy Approaches for Secondary Special Needs © Whurr Publishers Ltd 2002

CA3

Table 3.3 Science

Possible Classroom Problem	Possible Practical Approach	Further Advice via SENCO
	It may be necessary to seek advice from your SENCO in order to implement some of these approaches	Refer to gross motor skill sheet (**F1**)
Gross motor co-ordination		
■ Ability to maintain functional working position in:		
(a) sitting on high stool without back/foot support	■ Check sitting posture-stool/bench size and height, ensure adequate clearance for knees under bench and support for forearms Rest feet on stool crossbar for support to improve stability Consider science stool with back – arrange for REMAP to alter existing stools or buy alternative stool Allow student to re-establish posture by standing, stretching at agreed time intervals Consider working on an angled writing surface/clipboard	■ Refer to Occupational Therapy sheet (**OT1**) ■ Refer to Equipment resources (**ER**), Useful addresses ■ Refer to Equipment resources (**ER**)
(b) standing	■ Check bench height relative to student Provide adequate areas to 'prop' Provide benches which are height adjustable Ensure equipment for practical work is within reach Supply wooden platform for student if required, painted clearly for safety, e.g. bright yellow Consider allowing student to sit for part of practical work Interperse practical 'making' with 'designing' and recording	■ Refer to Occupational Therapy sheet (**OT1**) ■ Refer to Equipment resources (**ER**) ■ Refer to health and safety/ workshop regulations
■ Reduced stamina for extended periods of writing	■ Alternative recording methods, e.g. dictaphone, pre-prepared worksheets, appropriate ICT equipment Consider amanuensis Give realistic targets; set attainable goals Consider longer time to complete task Consider extra time allowance, fatigue breaks, adult support as a scribe in exam situations	■ Seek advice from ICT advisor, advisory teacher, occupational therapist and refer to Appendices (**A1** and **A3**) ■ Seek advice from educational pyschologist
■ Body awareness in practical group work	■ Undertake risk assessment Ensure adequate space to allow for uncoordinated movements Smaller groups for practical work Consider safety issues, raise student's awareness of the need to plan task methodically. Consider the need for adult support	■ Seek advice from school health and safety representative, refer to health and safety policy

Occupational Therapy Approaches for Secondary Special Needs © Whurr Publishers Ltd 2002

Table 3.3 Science

Possible Classroom Problem	Possible Practical Approach	Further Advice via SENCO
Gross motor co-ordination (continued)		
■ Mobility around the classroom	■ Heighten awareness of the need to maintain uncluttered aisles Reduce the number of students moving around the laboratory at any one time, e.g one group at a time Reduce student's need to move around the laboratory by collecting apparatus before starting Provide individual set of equipment	
■ Carrying and setting up potentially hazardous materials/equipment, e.g. test tubes, chemicals, tripod, glass containers, scalpels	■ Undertake risk assessment Enforce clear rules 'for the laboratory' Buddy working/adult support to carry equipment Analyse work area/space for safe and efficient use of equipment Use plastic basket for collecting items Use a temporary storage area for apparatus in use, e.g. 'in centre of table' Prioritize relevance of curricular task Enforce safety rules, e.g. wearing protective clothing	■ Seek advice from school health and safety representative, refer to school health and safety policy
■ Grading force of movement	■ Use more robust/larger containers Buddy working/adult support	
■ Participating in field trips	■ Consider safety implications and undertake risk assessment Consider buddy working/adult support	■ Refer to school field trips policy
Fine motor dexterity	**It may be necessary to seek advice from your SENCO in order to implement some of the approaches**	**Refer to fine motor dexterity skill sheet (F2)**
■ Reduced safety resulting from poorly controlled or impulsive movements	■ Undertake risk assessment Raise awareness of safety issues resulting from poor manual dexterity Consider providing classroom support Analyse work area/space to ensure safe and efficient use of equipment	■ Seek advice from health and safety representative/refer to school health and safety policy.

Occupational Therapy Approaches for Secondary Special Needs © Whurr Publishers Ltd 2002

CA3 **Science** (continued)

Possible Classroom Problem	Possible Practical Approach	Further Advice via SENCO
Fine motor dexterity (continued)		
■ Anchoring and stabilizing equipment	■ Use G clamps, non-slip mats Provide adult support	■ Refer to Equipment resources (**ER**)
■ Reduced tactile awareness which is further impaired by wearing gloves	■ Ensure gloves are the correct size Heighten teachers' awareness of student's difficulty	■ Refer to Equipment resources (**ER**) Seek advice from occupational therapist, advisory teachers
■ Handling and operating equipment, e.g. microscope, slides, circuit-boards, scalpels, tweezers, test tubes, pipettes, goggles	■ Consider stabilizing equipment with, e.g. dycem mat, clamp Trial alternative equipment Provide individual set of adapted equipment Provide part-prepared work to minimize necessity for fine precision movements Consider adult support/buddy working Undertake risk assessment Use ICT software to simulate experiment Ensure good lighting	■ Seek advice from school health and safety representative
■ Handling and measuring of materials, e.g. solids, liquids, due to poor fine motor control and reduced ability to grade pressure of movement	■ Use alternative measuring equipment which does not require as precise a movement Work with partner or adult when accuracy is paramount Use of ICT software to simulate experiment	
■ Recording evidence by handwriting	■ Check sitting posture-stool/bench size and height Consider adult support as an amanuensis Alternative recording methods, e.g. appropriate ICT, part-prepared worksheets Photocopy notes taken by group amanuensis	■ Refer to Occupational Therapy sheet (**OT1**) ■ Seek advice from ICT advisor, refer to Appendices (**A1** and **A3**)
drawing diagrams, tables, graphs, apparatus	■ Use appropriate ICT equipment, e.g. scanner, computer graphics Use commercially available stencils Provide part-prepared worksheets which only need to be labelled Provide adult support to produce drawings Allow student to trace from text books	■ Refer to Equipment resources (**ER**)
■ Reduced keyboard/mouse skills affecting ability to use ICT equipment	■ Provide sufficient forearm support – use wrist support/rest, appropriate size table Use a keyguard to improve accuracy Consider help to set up and carry equipment from class to class Trial alternative mouse devices and keyboards Use 'dampening' facility when key is depressed for too long	■ Refer to Equipment resources (**ER**)
■ Following health and safety procedures, e.g. putting on protective clothing/goggles/mask	■ Adapt fastenings, e.g. with velcro Consider adult/peer support	■ Seek advice from ICT advisor, advisory teacher, occupational therapist

Occupational Therapy Approaches for Secondary Special Needs © Whurr Publishers Ltd 2002

CA3 Science (continued)

CA3

Table 3.3 Science

Possible Classroom Problem	Possible Practical Approach	Further Advice via SENCO
Organizational skills	**It may be necessary to seek advice from your SENCO in order to implement some of these approaches**	**Refer to organizational skill sheet (F3) and Occupational Therapy sheet (OT7)**
■ Reduced health and safety awareness	■ Undertake risk assessment Use specific safety checklists Encourage student to pre-plan task, planning far enough ahead to anticipate problems Consider buddy working/adult support Ensure work area is uncluttered	■ Seek advice from school health and safety representative, refer to school health and safety policy
■ Organizing design process and performing practical tasks	■ Plan stages of task prior to starting Use checklists to show stage Use mind-mapping techniques Consider use of 'work schedules' Provide part-prepared experiments Consider 1:1 instruction on how to use specific equipment, e.g. microscope Give prompts and provide practical 'concrete' examples Reduce level of support as student makes progress	■ Refer to Further reading ■ Refer to Appendix (**A5**)
■ Presentation and layout of written work and experiments	■ Provide clear written methodology for experiments Use alternative recording methods e.g. part-prepared worksheets, stencils, appropriate ICT software Provide cue sheet showing sample layout Give concrete examples of expected positioning and layout Use lined/squared paper Parallel working with fellow student, adult support, buddy working	
■ Ability to follow verbal instructions	■ Reinforce with written notes/pictorial cue cards/diagrams depicting sequence to follow Give instructions in small steps and repeat instructions to ensure student has understood – give frequent recapping, e.g. 'what we have done', 'what we will do next' Consider adult support to ensure homework instructions are understood and written down, e.g. in homework diary	■ Seek advice from speech and language therapist
■ Remembering and sequencing formulas/equations	■ Give cue cards listing formulae/equations Break formulas/equations down and colour code sections	

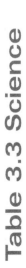

CA3 Science (continued)

Possible Classroom Problem	Possible Practical Approach	Further Advice via SENCO
Organizational skills (continued)		
■ Ability to e.g. follow written methodology	■ Break written instructions down into small steps, highlighting key points Provide combined written and diagrammatic/pictorial instructions Provide clear written methodology for experiments	
■ Impaired investigative skills, e.g. evaluating, analysing	■ Use mind-mapping techniques Use concrete examples to explain the process Reinforce general scientific principles	■ Refer to Further reading
■ Difficulty generalizing principles	■ Raise awareness of need to teach each individual stage of process as student will not automatically generalize concepts	
■ Negotiating self around laboratory to collect apparatus or to seek help	■ Ensure aisles are uncluttered Ensure student adequately pre-plans and collects all necessary equipment before starting task Heighten adult awareness to reduce need for student to leave task One group at a time to collect apparatus	■ Seek advice from school health & safety representative, refer to health & safety policy
Visual motor integration	**It may be necessary to seek advice from your SENCO in order to implement some of these approaches**	**Refer to visual motor integration skill sheet (F6)**
■ Inaccurate manipulative skills due to poor eye–hand co-ordination, e.g. using scissors, pipette, dissecting with scalpel	■ Choose activity carefully to enhance student's ability to succeed Reduce the need for accuracy by providing alternative equipment, e.g. enlarging container Adult support when accuracy paramount Check posture and optimize stability by resting elbows on bench, although this might not be possible when using some apparatus	■ Seek advice from occupational therapist, advisory teacher ■ Refer to Occupational Therapy sheet (**OT1**)
■ Neatness and presentation when recording evidence, e.g. writing, drawing	■ Use bullet points rather than full sentences Use alternative recording methods, e.g. appropriate ICT, stencils, part-prepared worksheets only needing to be labelled	■ Seek advice from ICT advisor, refer to Appendices (**A1** and **A3**)

CA3

Table 3.3 Science

Possible Classroom Problem	Possible Practical Approach	Further Advice via SENCO
Visual motor integration (continued)		
■ Neatness and presentation when recording evidence, e.g. writing, drawing	Allow student to trace apparatus from text book Provide lined/squared paper to help with layout Provide a proforma of suggested layout Use posters showing how to draw common equipment/apparatus Photocopy notes done by group scribe	
■ Use of microscope	■ Use alternatives, e.g. pre-prepared projector slides, OHP acetates Try enhancing work by linking microscope to computer Use adult support/buddy working to help set up microscope	
■ Construction tasks	■ Use alternative materials if possible, e.g. sturdy rather than flimsy Reduce the need for precision by using larger equipment Provide a part-prepared model Use adult support when accuracy is paramount	
Visual spatial relationships	**It may be necessary to seek advice from your SENCO in order to implement some of these approaches**	**Refer to visual spatial relationships skill sheet (F7)**
■ Using linear and vertical scanning	■ Reinforce working left to right, top to bottom and use of margin e.g. colour margin red or green, work to margin in book Use right-angled paper guide/clear perspex ruler as a line tracker Use squared and isometric paper to help placement	■ Refer to Foundation skill sheet (F5), Appendix (A4)
■ Drawing 2D representation of 3D objects	■ Work on squared/isometric paper Provide instructions on how to transfer 3D to 2D Teach 'rules' on how to draw common apparatus Draw for students, use stencils/templates	
■ Constructing 3D models	■ Give concrete example of completed model Complete part-made model Reproduce instructions so each stage of process is visually represented e.g. use photographs, pictures, line drawings depicting sequence of process Colour code initial 2D diagram to correspond with apparatus	■ Refer to Equipment resources (ER)

Possible Classroom Problem	Possible Practical Approach	Further Advice via SENCO
Visual spatial relationships (continued)		
■ Understanding scale – comparing the size of objects	■ Use graph paper as visual cue of size representation or use scale rule Use auditory cues and concrete examples of objects to assist comparison of scale	
■ Setting up experiments from 2D diagrams	■ Try using photographs/pictures/line drawings depicting sequence Use a base template to locate apparatus on working surface, e.g. pre-drawn plan for circuit Colour code initial 2D diagram to correspond with apparatus	
■ Presentation and layout for recording evidence	■ Use appropriate computer software, e.g. Clip Art™, scanner Use pre-drawn tables, diagrams, axis for graphs, highlighting data using different colours Use squared/graph paper Use line tracker/appropriate sized window/right-angled paper guide to help placement Provide proforma with suggested layout	■ Seek advice from ICT advisor ■ Refer to Equipment resources (**ER**)
■ Interpreting evidence	■ Use different colours to highlight categories of data Provide prompt sheet listing evidence to be gathered	
Visual figure ground discrimination	**It may be necessary to seek advice from your SENCO in order to implement some of these approaches**	**Refer to visual figure ground skill sheet (F9)**
■ Preparation for lesson in general	■ Limit the amount of information presented on page/board Limit the amount of copying from board or if essential use different colour chalks/pens to highlight key information Ensure work surfaces are clear Reinforce need to return equipment, e.g. burners, acids, scalpels to allocated storage area after use	
■ Drawing and interpreting data, graphs, tables and charts	■ Encourage student to highlight whilst working Use appropriate computer software, e.g. Clip Art™, scanner Use pre-drawn tables, diagrams, axis for graphs – highlighting key data using different colours Enlarge worksheets	■ Seek advice from ICT advisor

Possible Classroom Problem	Possible Practical Approach	Further Advice via SENCO
Visual figure ground discrimination (continued)		
■ Drawing and interpreting data, graphs, tables and charts	Use larger scale Limit the amount of information on each page, e.g. one graph on a page instead of four Use an appropriate-sized window e.g. to reduce visual information Use line tracker/right-angled paper guide to help scanning	■ Refer to Equipment resources (ER)
■ Reading and interpreting computer printouts Using and interpreting data sheets/lists	■ Use larger print to reduce amount of information on a sheet Use double-spaced print to reduce cluttered appearance Colour or highlight key information before lesson Encourage student to highlight whilst working Use appropriate-sized window e.g. to reduce visual information or a line tracker to help with scanning	■ Refer to Foundation skill sheet (F5), Appendix (A4)
■ Obtaining measurements, e.g. reading calibrations	■ Consider alternative equipment with clearer markings Alter position of equipment to find optimum visual acuity, e.g. elevating work, holding test tube against additional scale Ensure good contrast between substance and container/measuring jug	■ Refer to Equipment resources (ER) ■ Refer to Foundation skill sheet (F5)
■ Finding appropriate equipment, e.g. pipette, scalpel	■ Ensure items are stored correctly and clearly labelled	
■ Organization and layout of overlapping drawings	■ Use clear, uncluttered prepared worksheets to reduce need for drawing or allow student to trace from text book Consistent colour coding of equipment when copying or drawing Accentuate colour contrasts in practicals, e.g. work on a white surface, place white sheet behind work	
■ Cutting accurately, e.g. in dissections, to prepare microscope slides	■ Provide adult support when accuracy is paramount	
■ Multiple-choice questions within the same page	■ Highlight relevant part of question if it corresponds to several options Increase size of print and spacing – either by enlarging on photocopier or whilst drawing on computer Use of line tracker/appropriately sized window to reduce visual information	■ Refer to Equipment resources (ER)
■ Selecting correct part of written or diagrammatic instructions when a lot of information is presented on the same page	■ Reproduce instructions so each stage of the process is on separate sheets Colour code each stage of the process	

Occupational Therapy Approaches for Secondary Special Needs © Whurr Publishers Ltd 2002

CA3 Science (continued)

Possible Classroom Problem	Possible Practical Approach	Further Advice via SENCO
Visual form constancy	**It may be necessary to seek advice from your SENCO in order to implement some of these approaches**	**Refer to visual form constancy skill sheet (F8)**
■ Recognizing materials/objects in different forms to enable classification	■ Reinforce common properties of materials Give cue sheet listing common properties, e.g. a fish has gills and fins Provide concrete examples to manipulate and classify	
■ Making representative 3D models	■ Provide part or completed models	
■ Recognizing that the quantity is the same regardless of the shape of the container	■ Use a measuring device to demonstrate that the quantities are equal	
Visual closure	**It may be necessary to seek advice from your SENCO in order to implement some of these approaches**	**Refer to visual closure skill sheet (F10)**
■ Being able to see a complete formulas/life cycle/circuit	■ Use prompt cards to identify stages of the formulas/life cycle/circuit	
■ Identifying and locating objects on a crowded table/work bench when only part of the object is visible	■ Maintain clear/organized work surfaces	
■ Completing practical tasks, e.g. wiring a plug, setting up experiments, circuits, performing dissection, making models	■ Break down task and relate each stage to example of end product Make a series of visual cue cards identifying stages Work in 'parallel' with teacher	
■ Identifying and reproducing patterns	■ Adult support to discuss pattern Highlight elements/parts of pattern	

Table 3.3 Science

Possible Classroom Problem	Possible Practical Approach	Further Advice via SENCO
Visual memory/sequential memory	**It may be necessary to seek advice from your SENCO in order to implement some of these approaches**	**Refer to visual memory/sequential memory skill sheet (F11)**
■ Copying from the board/book	■ Reduce copying from board, e.g. use part-prepared work sheets or give own copy of board information Check student's position in e.g. class relative to board, position near and facing board Be aware of objects, in line of vision, which could interfere with student's view Try using different colours or stickers to differentiate sections of text to be copied.	■ Refer to Foundation skill sheet (F5)
■ Recording stages of the science process	■ Encourage student to take notes at each stage as they are working Take photographs of each stage	
■ Remembering formulas, symbols, and equations	■ Colour code categories of information, e.g. periodic table Provide cue card listing equations, formulas, symbols Talk through pattern Break equations/formulas down and colour code sections	
■ Remembering details of practical demonstrations	■ Break down each task and record stages, e.g. using digital camera, numbered pictorial cue cards Highlight each stage on instruction sheet Take notes during demonstrations, e.g. pictorial, prompt words	
Auditory processing and memory	**It may be necessary to seek advice from SENCO in order to implement some of these approaches**	**Refer to auditory processing and memory skill sheet (F12)**
■ Following and remembering verbal instructions	■ Give clear, concise instructions in small steps Repeat instructions, allowing student to verbalize back to check that she of he has heard and understood – frequent recapping Reinforce with written notes and visual cue cards Withdraw student to quiet area and give assistance Use a dictaphone	■ Seek advice from speech and language therapist

Possible Classroom Problem	Possible Practical Approach	Further Advice via SENCO
Auditory processing and memory (continued)		
■ Group discussion, e.g. ability to sift, summarize, use salient points, cite evidence	■ Frequent resumé of essential points by group leader Encourage student to record main points of discussion and write down any questions during discussion Ask student leading questions as a prompt Use mind-mapping techniques Allow student time to answer	■ Seek advice from educational psychologist, speech and language therapist ■ Refer to Further reading
■ Listening and responding in discussions	■ Give advance warning of forthcoming discussion Check position in class, e.g. sitting in front or facing speaker Use buddy/adult support Use pre-prepared cue cards	
■ Understanding scientific terminology	■ Use a glossary/cue cards listing terminology, apparatus names	
Social interaction	**It may be necessary to seek advice from your SENCO in order to implement some of these approaches**	**Refer to social interaction skill sheet (F13)**
■ Reluctance to handle certain material due to tactile sensitivity leading to an inappropriate response	■ Consider use of alternative materials Wear surgical gloves	
■ Awareness of personal space (own and others)	■ Social skills training programme Heighten teacher's and peers' awareness of student's difficulty	■ Seek advice from child and adolescent mental health service, educational psychologist
■ Impulsiveness	■ Heighten teacher's and peers' awareness to student's difficulty Allocate achievable tasks to student	
■ Working as part of a group	■ Consider adult facilitation Select group members carefully	

Occupational Therapy Approaches for Secondary Special Needs © Whurr Publishers Ltd 2002

Table 3.4 Design and technology

Possible Classroom Problem	Possible Practical Approach	Further Advice via SENCO
Gross motor co-ordination	**It may be necessary to seek advice from your SENCO in order implement some of these approaches**	**Refer to gross motor co-ordination skill sheet (F1)**
■ Ability to maintain functional working position and stamina when		
(a) sitting on chair or high stool without back/foot support	■ Check stool/chair, table/bench size and height Ensure adequate clearance for knees under bench and support for forearms Rest feet on crossbar for support to improve stability Consider stool with back or arrange for e.g. REMAP to alter existing stools Consider use of angled writing surface, e.g. clipboard, easel Allow child to re-establish posture by standing, stretching at agreed time intervals. Set attainable goals as output of work may be reduced	■ Refer to Occupational Therapy sheet (**OT1**) ■ Refer to Equipment resources (**ER**) and Useful addresses ■ Refer to Equipment resources (**ER**)
(b) standing	■ Check bench height and height of any machinery that student would need to access, e.g. pillar drill, scroll saws, acrylic wire bending equipment, etc. Provide benches which are adjustable Supply wooden platform if required, painted clearly for safety, e.g bright yellow Ensure equipment for practical work is within reach. Consider allowing student to have the option of sitting for part of practical work. Provide adequate areas to 'prop' Plan lesson so heavy physical work is undertaken early in lesson or intersperse practical 'making' with 'designing' and recording	■ Refer to Equipment resources (**ER**) ■ Refer to health and safety regulations/workshop regulations ■ Refer to health and safety regulations/workshop regulations
■ Reduced stamina for extended periods of writing therefore reduced output of work	■ Alternative recording methods, e.g. pre-prepared worksheets, notes, appropriate e.g. ICT, adult support as an amanuensis Encourage student to edit own work Give realistic targets; set attainable goals Consider longer time to complete task	■ Seek advice from ICT advisor, refer to Appendices (**A1** and **A3**)

Possible Classroom Problem	Possible Practical Approach	Further Advice via SENCO

Gross motor co-ordination (continued)

Possible Classroom Problem	Possible Practical Approach	Further Advice via SENCO
■ Body awareness in practical group work	■ Undertake risk assessment Ensure adequate space to allow for uncoordinated movements Consider smaller groups for practical work Consider safety issues, raise student's awareness of the need to plan task methodically Consider the need for adult support	■ Seek advice from school health and safety representative, refer to health and safety regulations
■ Mobility around the classroom	■ Heighten awareness of the need to maintain uncluttered aisles Reduce the number of students moving around the room/workshop at any one time – enforce clear rules 'for the room' Reduce the student's need to move around the room/workshop by collecting equipment before starting task Provide individual set of equipment Use temporary storage for equipment in use in 'tool well' or centre of table to ensure tools are not knocked off table	
■ Carrying and setting up potentially dangerous equipment, e.g. scissors, saws, knives, clamps, hot saucepans	■ Undertake risk assessment Buddy working/adult support to carry equipment in workshop Consider alternative means of carrying/moving equipment Prioritize relevance of curricular task for student Analyse work area/space for safe and efficient use of equipment Recognize certain skills need to be 'taught' not 'caught', e.g. when using craft knives use safety rulers and cutting mats Observe correct lifting procedures Motor programme to improve strength	■ Seek advice from school health and safety representative, refer to school health and safety policy, school manual handling policy
■ Grading force of movements	■ Choose materials of appropriate density/resistance Seek alternative medium – refer to curriculum requirements Buddy working/adult support	■ Refer to Occupational Therapy sheet (**OT6**)

CA4 Design and technology (continued)

Table 3.4 Design and technology

Possible Classroom Problem	Possible Practical Approach	Further Advice via SENCO
Fine motor dexterity	**It may be necessary to seek advice from your SENCO in order to implement some of these approaches**	**Refer to fine motor dexterity skill sheet (F2)**
■ Reduced safety resulting from poorly controlled or impulsive movements	■ Undertake risk assessment Raise the student's awareness of safety issues Consider adult support/buddy working Prioritize relevance of curricular tasks for student Ensure workspace/area is uncluttered Motor programme to improve hand/body strength	■ Seek advice from school health and safety representative, refer to school health and safety policy ■ Refer to Occupational Therapy sheets (**OT5** and **OT6**)
■ Handling and operating equipment, e.g. sewing machine, vices, lathe, saw, food mixer, knives, jigs, milling machine, digital camera	■ Consider stabilizing equipment, e.g. use dycem mat, clamp Consider providing part-prepared work to minimize necessity for fine precision movements Trial alternative equipment Provide individual set of adapted equipment Use of specialist equipment Ensure good lighting Consider adult support/buddy working	■ Refer to Equipment resources (**ER**) ■ Seek advice from occupational therapist advisory teacher
■ Handling and measuring materials (e.g. solids, liquids) due to reduced ability to grade pressure of movement	■ Use alternative measuring equipment which allows for imprecise movements Work with partner or adult when accuracy is paramount	

■ Recording evidence by
  handwriting
  drawing diagrams, tables, graphs, apparatus
	■ Check sitting posture
	Alternative recording methods e.g. adult support as an amanuensis, appropriate ICT, digital/video camera, part prepared worksheets
	Adult support to produce drawings for student
	Use commonly available stencils
	Allow student to trace diagram, table from text book
		■ Refer to Occupational Therapy sheet (**OT1**)
		■ Seek advice from ICT advisor, refer to Appendices (**A1** and **A3**)
		
		■ Refer to Equipment resources (**ER**)

■ Reduced keyboard or mouse skills affecting ability to use ICT equipment	■ Provide sufficient forearm support – use appropriate chair and table, use a wrist rest/support Try keyguard to increase accuracy Consider adult support help to set up and carry equipment Use alternative mouse devices and keyboards Use 'dampening' facility to reduce repetition when key is depressed for too long	■ Refer to Appendix (**A3**) and Equipment resources (**ER**) ■ Refer to Equipment resources (**ER**) ■ Refer to ICT advisor, advisory teacher, occupational therapist

Possible Classroom Problem	Possible Practical Approach	Further Advice via SENCO
Fine motor dexterity (continued)		
■ Reduced tactile awareness which is further impaired by wearing gloves e.g. handling hot plastics/metals, etc.	■ Ensure gloves are the correct size Heighten teachers' awareness of student's difficulties Consider safety implications and undertake risk assessment	■ Refer to school health and safety policy, seek advice from health and safety representative
■ Following health and safety procedures, e.g. putting on goggles, gloves, aprons	■ Peer/adult support to ensure equipment fitted adequately Adapt fastenings, e.g. with velcro	■ Refer to Equipment resources (**ER**), seek advice from school health and safety representative, occupational therapist
■ Anchoring and stabilizing equipment	■ Use G clamps, belly clamp, spiked board, non-slip mat, jig or similar stabilization Provide adult support	
Organizational skills	**It may be necessary to seek advice from your SENCO in order to implement some of these approaches**	**Refer to organizational skill sheet (F3) and Occupational Therapy sheet (OT7)**
■ Reduced health and safety awareness	■ Undertake risk assessments Use safety checklists Encourage student to pre-plan task, planning far enough ahead to anticipate problems which they will encounter/have to overcome Teacher input may be needed to help with problem or steer student towards easier route/outcome Consider buddy working/adult support Ensure work area is uncluttered	■ Seek advice from school health and safety representative, refer to school health and safety policy
■ Spatial awareness problems	■ Restrict working areas around key machinery Reinforce floor markings/safety areas/rules for personal space Encourage students to work in same area each week to build up familiarity with immediate surroundings	
■ Organizing design process and performing practical tasks	■ Plan stages of task prior to starting Use mind-mapping techniques Use checklists to show stages Consider use of 'work schedules' Use of part-prepared work	■ Refer to Further reading ■ Refer to Appendix (**A5**)

CA4 Design and technology (continued)

Table 3.4 Design and technology

Possible Classroom Problem	Possible Practical Approach	Further Advice via SENCO
Organizational skills (continued)		
■ Organizing design process and performing practical tasks (continued)	■ Consider 1:1 instruction on use of specific equipment, e.g. lathe, sewing machine, food mixer, jigsaw Give prompts/provide practical concrete examples as design is by nature 'abstract' so it may be difficult for student to assimulate what is required of them	
■ Ability to follow verbal instructions	■ Reinforce with diagrams/written notes/pictorial cue cards depicting sequence to follow Give instructions in small steps and repeat to ensure student has understood Provide frequent recapping – 'what we have done; what we will do next' Consider use of 'work schedules' Adult support to ensure homework instructions are understood and written down, e.g. in homework diary	■ Refer to Appendix (**A5**)
■ Ability to follow written methodology	■ Break written instructions down into small steps, highlighting key points Provide combined written and diagrammatic instructions	
■ Presentation and layout of written work and practical processes	■ Use alternative recording methods, e.g. part-prepared worksheets, stencils and appropriate ICT Use of squared/graph paper/guidelines Parallel working or adult support Place student so left- or right-handed students are not colliding Use 'writing frame' and give cue sheet or concrete examples suggesting layout for work	■ Seek advice from ICT advisor, refer to Appendices (**A1** and **A3**) ■ Refer to Further reading
■ Impaired investigative skills, e.g. evaluating, analysing, 'disassembly' – may prove difficult where component parts are small	■ Use mind-mapping techniques Use concrete examples to explain the process	■ Refer to Further reading
■ Difficulty generalizing principles	■ Raise awareness of need to teach each individual stage of process as student will not automatically generalize concept	■ Seek advice from educational psychologist
■ Using ICT equipment	■ Diagramatic step-by-step guide on how to set up equipment Cue cards for use of Internet or specific signature, e.g. CAD, CAM	■ Seek advice from ICT advisor, advisory teacher

Occupational Therapy Approaches for Secondary Special Needs © Whurr Publishers Ltd 2002

CA4 Design and technology (continued)

Possible Classroom Problem	Possible Practical Approach	Further Advice via SENCO
Organizational skills (continued)		
■ Negotiating self around work area to collect equipment	■ Position tables/benches to allow for safe movement of individuals with equipment, e.g. 'one group at a time to collect' Ensure aisles are uncluttered Adequate pre-planning to ensure student has necessary equipment before starting Give student a choice to self-collect equipment, work with a partner or ask an adult to collect on their behalf	■ Refer to school health and safety representative/policy
Visual motor integration	**It may be necessary to seek advice from your SENCO in order to implement some of these approaches**	**Refer to visual motor integration skill sheet (F6)**
■ Accurate manipulative skills due to poor eye–hand co-ordination e.g. using scissors, saw, knife, needle	■ Choose activity carefully to enhance student's ability to succeed Adult support when accuracy paramount Check posture and ensure stability with elbows resting on bench, although this may not be possible when using machinery/tools Use of aids, e.g. needle threaders or cutting jigs and templates	
■ Neatness, presentation, accurate placement of parts when drawing	■ Use of part-prepared work Use computer software Explore properties of finished product prior to drawing Discuss properties of component parts in relation to the whole Use stencils, templates Allow student to trace from text book	■ Refer to Equipment resources (**ER**) ■ Seek advice from ICT advisor
■ Neatness and presentation of handwriting	■ Use alternative recording methods, e.g. dictaphone, appropriate ICT, provide notes and worksheets to reduce the amount of copying Use bullet points rather than full sentence construction Use 'writing frames' Use appropriate lined paper to help with letter placement or 'underlays' so guidelines can be seen through paper Use clipboards/paper clips to keep papers together and still Photocopy notes done by group scribe – shared by all	■ Seek advice from ICT advisor, refer to Appendices (**A1** and **A3**) ■ Refer to Further reading

CA4 Design and technology (continued)

Table 3.4 Design and technology

Possible Classroom Problem	Possible Practical Approach	Further Advice via SENCO
Visual motor integration (continued)		
Neatness and presentation of handwriting (continued)	Consider allowing longer time to complete task or ask peer/group member or adult to scribe Consider extra time allowance or adult support as a scribe in exam situations	Seek advice from educational pyschologist
Construction tasks	Use of alternative materials, e.g. sturdy rather than flimsy – refer to curricular requirements Reduce need for precision by using larger equipment Provide part-prepared model Use adult support when accuracy is paramount	
Visual spatial relationships	**It may be necessary to seek advice from your SENCO before implementing some of these approaches**	**Refer to visual spatial relationships skill sheet (F7)**
Using linear and vertical scanning	Reinforce working left to right, top to bottom and use of margin, e.g. colour margin red or green, work to margin in book Use right-angled paper guide Use clear perspex ruler as a line tracker Use squared and isometric paper to help placing and 3D drawings	Refer to Foundation skill sheet (**F5**), Appendix (**A4**)
Selecting correct part of diagramatic instruction when a lot of information presented on same page	Reproduce instructions so each stage of the process is on separate sheet Colour code each stage	
Drawing 2D representation of 3D objects	Work on squared or isometric paper Provide instructions on how to transfer 3D to 2D and vice versa Teach 'rules' on how to draw common objects Draw for students and/or use stencils/templates	
Constructing 3D models	Give concrete examples of completed model Complete part-made model Make trial model from card or paper first Reproduce instructions so each stage of process is visually represented	

Possible Classroom Problem	Possible Practical Approach	Further Advice via SENCO
Visual spatial relationships (continued)		
■ Constructing 3D models (continued)	Try using photographs/pictures/line drawing depicting sequence of process as per 'Lego technic' cards Colour code initial 2D diagram to correspond with apparatus Reinforce spatial orientation on model or plans	■ Refer to Equipment resources (**ER**)
■ Understanding scale – comparing the size of objects	■ Use isometric paper/graph paper to assist 'scaling' process Keep scale simple, e.g. 2:1, 3:1, 4:1 Use graph paper or scale ruler as visual cue of size representation Use auditory cues and concrete examples of objects to assist comparison of scale	
■ Presentation and layout of work	■ Use appropriate computer software, e.g. Clip Art™, scanner Use pre-drawn tables, diagrams, axis for graphs, highlight data using different colours. Provide proforma with suggested layout	■ Refer to Equipment resources (**ER**)
■ Presentation and layout for practical projects	■ Provide proforma with suggested layout Use line tracker/window/right-angled paper guide to help placement Use graph/square paper to assist with correct placement of parts Reinforce spatial orientation of component parts Draw scaled template to use as point of reference	
Visual figure ground discrimination	**It may be necessary to seek advice from your SENCO in order to implement some of these approaches**	**Refer to visual figure ground skill sheet (F9)**
■ Preparation for lesson in general	■ Ensure work surfaces are clear Reinforce need to return equipment, e.g. pens, saw, cooking equipment to allocated storage area after use or end of lesson Limit the amount of information on a page/board Limit the amount of copying from board or if essential use different colour chalks/pens to highlight key information Produce worksheet with key information already typed on it	

Table 3.4 Design and technology

Possible Classroom Problem	Possible Practical Approach	Further Advice via SENCO
Visual figure ground discrimination (continued)		
■ Preparation for lesson in general (continued)	■ Reduce clutter on table or board Consider use of 'work schedules'	■ Refer to Appendix (**A5**)
■ Drawing and interpreting data, graphs, tables and charts	■ Encourage student to highlight whilst working Use pre-drawn tables, diagrams with axis highlighted in different colours or key data highlighted Use line tracker/appropriate sized window/right-angle paper guide to help scanning Use larger scale Limit the amount of information on each page, e.g one table on a page instead of four tables Use appropriate computer software, e.g. Clip Art™, scanner	■ Refer to Equipment resources (**ER**)
■ Reading and interpreting computer printouts Using and interpreting data sheets/lists	■ Use large print to reduce information on a sheet Use double-spaced print to reduce cluttered appearance Colour or highlight key information before lesson Look at 'font' in terms of readability Encourage student to highlight whilst working Use appropriate-sized window or a line tracker to reduce visual field	■ Refer to Equipment resources (**ER**)
■ Obtaining measurements, e.g. reading calibrations	■ Consider alternative equipment with clearer markings/calibrations Alter position of equipment to find optimum visual acuity, e.g. elevating work Ensure good contrast between material and measuring tool, e.g. magnifying glass, ruler, measuring jug, weighing scales	■ Refer to Foundation skill sheet (**F5**), Appendix (**A4**)
■ Multiple-choice questions within the same page	■ Highlight relevant part of question if it corresponds to several options Increase size of print and spacing – either by enlarging on photocopier or whilst drawing up on computer Use line tracker/appropriate sized windows to reduce visual information	■ Refer to Equipment resources (**ER**)

Occupational Therapy Approaches for Secondary Special Needs © Whurr Publishers Ltd 2002

CA4 Design and technology (continued)

Possible Classroom Problem	Possible Practical Approach	Further Advice via SENCO
Visual figure ground discrimination (continued)		
■ Organization and layout of overlapping drawings	■ Use clear, uncluttered part-prepared worksheets to limit drawing Consistent colour coding of equipment when copying or drawing Accentuate colour contrast in practical work, e.g. work on a white board	
■ Finding appropriate item, e.g. screw, spoon, blade from pot/drawer/tray	■ Ensure items are stored correctly and clearly labelled Provide surface which gives good contrast to assist with sorting/finding Protect sharp knives, etc. when kept in drawers rather then knife rack	
■ Finding appropriate equipment for use	■ Use of shadow board for storing equipment Ensure only essential equipment on bench/table	
■ Cutting materials accurately, e.g. seeing line on material	■ Draw thicker/darker line in contrasting colour Provide template in contrasting colour to cut around Provide safety ruler or similar jig/specialist equipment to assist the cutting process Provide adult support when accuracy is paramount	
■ Selecting correct guideline on pattern	■ Highlight appropriate line to assist student with cutting	
Visual form constancy	**It may be necessary to seek advice from your SENCO in order to implement some of these approaches**	**Refer to form constancy skill sheet (F8)**
■ Recognizing the quantity is the same regardless of shape of container/size of container	■ Use a measuring device to demonstrate that the quantities are equal	
■ Understanding and generalizing the common properties of an object/utensil/plan, e.g. a spoon is still a spoon regardless of size, material, orientation	■ Use cue cards listing essential properties Discuss common properties of object/utensil and provide concrete examples	

CA4 Design and technology (continued)

Table 3.4 Design and technology

Possible Classroom Problem	Possible Practical Approach	Further Advice via SENCO
Visual form constancy (continued)		
■ Investigating and classifying a variety of design styles and traditions	■ Heighten teacher's awareness of student's difficulties Provide checklist listing common properties	
■ Making representative 3D models	■ Provide part or completed models	
■ Drawing 2D shapes in different orientations on grid	■ Use appropriate ICT software, e.g. clipart™ Work on squared paper or isometric paper Instruct student on how to change orientation of shape by using concrete examples Use stickers, stencils, templates to assist with orientation	
Visual closure	**It may be necessary to seek advice from your SENCO in order to implement some of these approaches**	**Refer to visual closure skill sheet (F10)**
■ Being able to visualize completed product	■ Use prompt cards/pictorial representation to identify each stage of the process Talk through each step of the process in relation to finished project, 'Here's one I've done earlier'	
■ Identifying/locating objects on crowded workbench when only part of object is visible	■ Maintain clear, organized work surfaces	
■ Practical tasks, e.g. making a cake, woodwork, projects, sewing a garment	■ Break down task and relate each stage to an example of end product. Make a series of visual cue cards identifying stages – especially important when following prescribed tasks, e.g. recipes Work 'parallel' with teacher, i.e. teacher 'does'/student 'does'; teachers performs next task/student copies, etc.	

Possible Classroom Problem	Possible Practical Approach	Further Advice via SENCO
visual memory/sequential memory	**It may be necessary to seek advice from your SENCO in order to implement some of these approaches**	**Refer to visual memory/sequential memory skill sheet (F11)**
Copying from the board/book	■ Reduce copying from board, e.g. use part-prepared work sheets or give own copy of board information Check student's position in class relative to board; position near and facing board Be aware of objects, in line of vision, which could affect student's view Ask teacher to use different colours to differentiate sections of text to be copied Use stickers on board as visual marker Give adequate time for student to record work	■ Refer to Foundation skill sheet **(F5)**
Remembering details of practical demonstration	■ Teach note-taking techniques Take notes during demonstration, e.g. pictorial shorthand, prompt words Use numbered pictorial cue cards Break down each task and record stages of process using digital camera, etc. Use of writing frames/headings as memory cues, e.g. items to collect, ingredients, method, finished product Highlight each stage if needed	■ Refer to Further reading
Recording stages of process for construction	■ Encourage student to take notes of each stage as they are working Take photographs of each stage	
Auditory processing and memory	**It may be necessary to seek advice from your SENCO in order to implement some of these approaches**	**Refer to auditory processing and memory skill sheet (F12)**
Following and remembering verbal instructions	■ Use other senses to support auditory sense Use dictaphone Give clear, concise instructions in small steps Repeat instructions and allow student to verbalize back to check that they have heard and understood Reinforce with written notes or sequential diagrams Withdraw student to quiet area and give assistance	■ Seek advice from speech and language therapist

CA4

Table 3.4 Design and technology

Possible Classroom Problem	Possible Practical Approach	Further Advice via SENCO
Auditory processing and memory (continued)		
■ Group discussion, e.g. ability to sift, summarize, use salient points, cite evidence	■ Frequent resumé of essential points by group leader Encourage student to record main points of discussion and write down any questions during discussion Ask student leading questions as a prompt Use mind-mapping techniques Allow time for student to answer	■ Seek advice from educational psychologist, speech and language therapist ■ Refer to Further reading
■ Listening and responding in discussions	■ Give advance warning of forthcoming discussion Check position in class, e.g. sitting in front or facing speaker Use buddy working/adult support Use pre-prepared cue cards	
■ Understanding relevant terminology	■ Use of glossary/cue cards	
Social interaction	**It may be necessary to seek advice from your SENCO in order to implement some of these approaches**	**Refer to social interaction skill sheet (F13)**
■ Low self-esteem leading to withdrawal	■ Build student's confidence by breaking down task Appropriate/fair use of praise and reward	
■ Reluctance to handle certain material due to tactile sensitivity leading to inappropriate response	■ Consider use of alternative methods Wear surgical gloves	
■ Impulsiveness	■ Undertake risk assessment Heighten teacher's and peers' awareness of student's difficulty Select group members carefully Ensure student has uncluttered work area Consider adult facilitation	■ Refer to school health and safety representative
■ Reduced awareness of personal space (own and others)	■ Social skills programme Heighten peers' and teachers' awareness of student's difficulty	
■ Working as part of group	■ Select group members carefully/consider adult facilitation Allocate alternative task to student	

Table 3.5 Information communication technology (ICT)

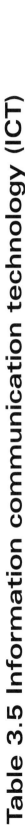

Possible Classroom Problem	Possible Practical Approach	Further Advice via SENCO
Gross motor co-ordination	**It may be necessary to seek advice from your SENCO in order to implement some of these approaches**	**Refer to gross motor skill sheet (F1)**
■ Ability to maintain functional typing position	■ Check sitting posture – chair/table size, height Provide chair with footrest if feet not on floor or stool with low back support and crossbar Ensure office chair is height adjusted and has brakes Raise supports at the rear of the keyboard to angle board or place on an angled surface if a greater angle is required Provide rise and fall computer table	■ Refer to Occupational Therapy sheet (**OT1**) and Appendix (**A3**) ■ Refer to Equipment resources (**ER**)
Fine motor dexterity	**It may be necessary to seek advice from your SENCO in order to implement some of these approaches**	**Refer to fine motor dexterity skill sheet (F2)**
■ Fluency and speed for keyboard skills	■ Check optimum supportive working posture is used Practise keyboard skills to improve fluency Colour code keyboard – sticky letters are available in colours especially black on yellow Try a keyguard to improve accuracy Try 'dampening keys' to reduce repetition when key is depressed for too long – on a PC go to control panel and select keyboard, then change the rate of repeat keys to slow and apply Try big keyed keyboard as it allows the student to hold down the key without a repeat	■ Refer to Appendix (**A3**) ■ Refer to Equipment resources ■ Seek advice from ICT advisor
■ Precise mouse control	■ Consider alternative equipment, e.g. rollerball, joystick, mouse devices	■ Seek advice from ICT advisor
■ Limited fine motor ability	■ Consider alternative equipment, e.g. voice-activated systems, mouse devices, switches, big keyed keyboard Consider adult/peer support	■ Seek advice from ICT advisor and Appendix (**A3**)

Table 3.5 Information communication technology (ICT)

Possible Classroom Problem	Possible Practical Approach	Further Advice via SENCO
Organizational skills	**It may be necessary to seek advice from your SENCO in order to implement some of these approaches**	**Refer to organizational skill sheet (F3)**
Layout of work	Create and use appropriate templates Consistent use of different type size, fonts, etc., by setting as a default Encourage regular editing of work Provide peer/adult support Mind-mapping software	Seek advice from ICT advisor
Systematic analysis of information	Organize information clearly on cue cards	
Ability to solve problems	Reinforce analytical processes	
Re-organizing information and presenting information in different formats	Provide concrete examples showing a range of formats	
Using database and spreadsheets	Give clear instructions, reinforced with written/diagrammatic cues Encourage appropriate pre-planning Use mind-mapping techniques Clarify expectations prior to student starting	Refer to Further reading Refer to Appendix (A5)
Designing information systems and evaluating existing systems, e.g. evaluating a website	Breakdown requirements/process Give key points for evaluating information	
Ability to follow written methodology	Encourage student to print instructions	
Using computer software, e.g. finding way around computer	Use small filing/index cards, laminated sheets for easy reference Provide adult/peer support	
Visual motor integration	**It may be necessary to seek advice from your SENCO in order to implement some of these approaches**	**Refer to visual motor integration skill sheet (F6)**
Depressing correct key	Reinforce keyboard/touch typing skills Try using a key guard to improve accuracy Trial alternative keyboards	Refer to Equipment resources and Appendix (A3)
Accurate mouse control	Use alternative mouse devices, e.g. with dampener	Seek advice from ICT advisor

Occupational Therapy Approaches for Secondary Special Needs © Whurr Publishers Ltd 2002

CA5 ICT (continued)

Possible Classroom Problem	Possible Practical Approach	Further Advice via SENCO
Visual spatial relationships	**It may be necessary to seek advice from your SENCO in order to implement some of these approaches**	**Refer to visual spatial relationships skill sheet (F7)**
■ Using linear and vertical scanning	■ Try double spacing of text by setting in default Try 'lined' screens Try using a range of fonts or colours to help differentiate sections Enlarge information on the screen Use software with an automatic scan, e.g. Clicker 4 or Writing with Symbols 2000 version.	■ Refer to Foundation skill sheet (F5) and Appendices (A3 and A4) ■ Refer to ICT advisor
■ Recognizing uniformity or differences in font size	■ Use on screen editing facility	
■ Interpreting and producing a range of layouts e.g. spreadsheets, posters	■ Use templates and tab settings Adult support to set tab settings and encourage student to regularly check that settings have not moved Discuss key features of layout Try using colours to help differentiate section/columns	
■ Understanding and using 3D representation of objects on the screen	■ Provide a concrete example of object for student to manipulate Compare screen image with concrete example	
■ Recognizing that several windows are open on the desktop	■ Encourage dragging to separate windows Minimize or close unused windows	
Visual figure ground discrimination	**It may be necessary to seek advice from your SENCO in order to implement some of these approaches**	**Refer to visual figure ground skill sheet (F9)**
■ Fluency for reading information presented in different font styles and sizes	■ Ensure font style and size are as consistent as possible Identify which font styles/sizes are more easily recognized – set these up in control panel and user on the PC	
■ Understanding and interpreting information presented in computer graphics when orientation is altered	■ Talk through changes in orientation by slowly demonstrating movements on screen or using concrete examples	
■ Identifying relevant information on the screen when lots of irrelevant information is presented, e.g. internet pages	■ Try to reduce information on the screen e.g. remove drawings from site	■ Refer to Foundation skill sheet (F5)

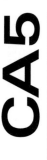

Table 3.5 Information communication technology (ICT)

Possible Classroom Problem	Possible Practical Approach	Further Advice via SENCO
Visual figure ground discrimination (continued)		
■ Identifying relevant information on the screen when lots of irrelevant information is presented, e.g. internet pages	■ Try selecting internet sites that only display information in a simple way, e.g. text-based screens Try using paper/acetate overlays with apertures on screen to reduce visual information	
■ Recognizing that several windows are open at once on the desktop	■ Adult/peer support to raise student's awareness Encourage use of dragging to reduce overlapping	
■ Locating cursor on the screen	■ Ensure good contrast between cursor and screen Use a more visually distinctive cursor	
■ Locating specific icons, tools	■ Heighten staff awareness of student's difficulty	
Visual closure	**It may be necessary to seek advice from your SENCO in order to implement some of these approaches**	**Refer to visual closure skill sheet (F10)**
■ Awareness that the information visible on the screen is only part of the work on the page	■ Encourage student to scan whole document regularly by using scroll bars Use the whole page preview function	
■ Recognizing that several windows are open when only parts of the windows are visible	■ Encourage dragging to separate windows	
Visual memory/sequential memory	**It may be necessary to seek advice from your SENCO in order to implement some of these approaches**	**Refer to visual memory/sequential memory skill sheet (F11)**
■ Remembering content of information on previous windows	■ Encourage awareness of the need regularly to check previous information Print off previous information Encourage note-taking of key information	
■ Remembering route taken in an internet search	■ Encourage use of 'history' function Encourage use of 'back' and 'forward' functions Set up effective filing system for 'favourites'	

Occupational Therapy Approaches for Secondary Special Needs © Whurr Publishers Ltd 2002

Possible Classroom Problem	Possible Practical Approach	Further Advice via SENCO
Visual memory/sequential memory (continued)		
■ Remembering work in progress when it is no longer visible on screen	■ Encourage student to scan whole documents regularly Use whole page function	
■ Remembering the function of icons, tools	■ Provide a cue card listing functions	
■ Remembering correct sequence when using pathways, e.g. to open a file	■ Provide cue card listing sequence, with visual prompts	
Auditory processing and memory	**It may be necessary to seek advice from your SENCO in order to implement some of these approaches**	**Refer to auditory processing and memory skill sheet (F12)**
■ Following and remembering verbal instruction	■ Give clear, concise instructions in small steps Repeat instructions and allow student to verbalize back to ensure student has understood Reinforce instructions with written/diagrammatic notes Use dictaphone Use mind-mapping software	
■ Group discussions, ability to sift and summarize	■ Write down key words to act as reminders	■ Seek advice from ICT advisor
Social interaction		**Refer to social interaction skill sheet (F13)**
■ Participating in group work	■ Provide adult support Carefully consider student's role in group work	

Table 3.6 History

CA6

Possible Classroom Problem	Possible Practical Approach	Further Advice via SENCO
	It may be necessary to seek advice from your SENCO in order to implement some of these approaches	**Refer to gross motor skill sheet (F1)**
Gross motor co-ordination		
■ Ability to maintain e.g. functional writing posture	■ Check sitting posture – chair/table size and height Consider working on an angled surface, e.g. clipboard, lever-arch file Consider rise and fall table with tilting surface	■ Refer to Occupational Therapy sheet (**OT1**) and Equipment resources (**ER**) ■ Refer to Equipment resources (**ER**)
■ Stamina for extended periods of writing Reduced quantity of written work, which will include completion of homework	■ Alternative recording methods, e.g. dictaphone, appropriate ICT, voice-activated computer software, part-prepared worksheets Consider adult support an amenuensis Encouraging editing of work Bullet points rather than sentence construction, e.g. use 'writing frames' Give realistic targets – set attainable goals Allow student to re-establish posture by standing, stretching, etc. at agreed time intervals, i.e 15 minutes Consider extending time to complete task Consider extra time allowance and fatigue breaks in exam Record homework using dictaphone/tape recorder for transcribing later Attend homework club (arranged by SENCO) if student is not too tired	■ Seek advice from ICT advisor, refer to Appendices (**A1** and **A3**) ■ Refer to Further reading ■ Seek advice from educational psychologist
■ Mobility around the classroom	■ Identify safe route to avoid bags, feet, etc. Keep pathways as clear as possible clear Review position in class – consider sitting at end of row/table or near aisle	
■ Participating in field trips, expeditions, e.g. museums	■ Consider safety implications, undertake risk assessment Consider buddy working/adult support	■ Refer to school field trips policy
■ Stamina and standing tolerance when on field trips	■ Use of fold-up shooting sticks for rest periods Provide piece of waterproof fabric to sit on Choose group members carefully	■ Refer to Equipment resources (**ER**)

CA6 History (continued)

Possible Classroom Problem | Possible Practical Approach | Further Advice via SENCO

Possible Classroom Problem	Possible Practical Approach	Further Advice via SENCO
Fine motor dexterity	**It may be necessary to seek advice from your SENCO in order to implement some of these approaches**	**Refer to fine motor dexterity skill sheet (F2)**
■ Neatness of handwriting and presentation of work	■ Check sitting posture – chair/table size and height Use lined paper to help with letter placement Consider alternative recording methods, e.g. appropriate ICT, part-prepared worksheets Consider adult support an amenuensis	■ Refer to Occupational Therapy sheet (**OT1**) ■ Seek advice from ICT advisor, refer to Appendices (**A1** and **A3**)
■ Fluency and speed of handwriting	■ Check sitting posture – chair/table size and height Accept that quantity of work will be reduced Consider alternative pencil grasps and trial different writing tools Consider adult support an amenuensis Encourage pressure awareness – consider paper texture Consider alternative methods of recording, e.g. dictaphone, appropriate part-prepared worksheets	■ Refer to Occupational Therapy sheets (**OT1** and **OT3**) and Equipment resources (**ER**) ■ Seek advice from ICT advisor, refer to Appendices (**A1** and **A3**)
■ Submitting incomplete homework	■ Record work on dictaphone for transcribing later Provide part-prepared notes and worksheets Consider student's difficulties when setting homework	
■ Using ICT equipment due to reduced keyboard and mouse skills	■ Consider adult support to set up and carry equipment from class to class Provide sufficient forearm support – use appropriate-sized table and wrist rest/support Teach keyboard/touch typing skills Colour code keys on keyboard Try alternative mouse devices and keyboards Use 'dampening' facility to reduce repetition when key is depressed for too long Use a keyguard to improve accuracy	■ Refer to Equipment resources (**ER**) ■ Seek advice from ICT advisor, refer to Appendix (**A3**) ■ Refer to Equipment resources (**ER**)
■ Using instruments, e.g. ruler, scissors	■ Trial alternative different equipment Consider buddy working/adult support	■ Refer to Equipment resources (**ER**)

Table 3.6 History

Possible Classroom Problem	Possible Practical Approach	Further Advice via SENCO
Fine motor dexterity (continued)		
■ Drawing accurate maps, diagrams and graphs	■ Provide stencils, templates Use appropriate ICT software, e.g. computer graphics, Clip Art™ Provide pre-prepared/part-prepared worksheets Allow student to trace from text book	
■ Model making	■ Consider alternative materials, e.g. foam Use velcro, pre-cut templates Consider buddy working /adult support	
Organizational skills	**It may be necessary to seek advice from your SENCO in order to implement some of these approaches**	**Refer to organizational skill sheet (F3)**
■ Chronological understanding and the concept of passing of time	■ Use concrete examples to help reinforce time sequences, e.g. time line	■ Seek advice from educational pyschologist
■ Ability to follow verbal instructions	■ Reinforce with written notes Give instructions in small steps and repeat instructions Ask student to repeat instructions back to check they have heard and understood If possible withdraw to quiet area and give assistance Provide assistance to ensure homework instructions are understood – use homework diary	■ Seek advice from speech and language therapist
■ Ability to follow written instructions	■ Break down instructions into small steps Write instructions in point form, underline/highlight key instructions Withdraw to quiet area and give assistance Consider buddy working/adult support	
■ Organizing thought process to express clearly historical events in context	■ Give prompts (verbal or written) Ask leading questions Use mind-mapping techniques Allow student time to answer	■ Seek advice from educational psychologist ■ Refer to Further reading
■ Selecting appropriate information, e.g. written text, maps, plans	■ Provide cue card listing what to look for in text, maps, etc. Use highlighters/colour coding systems Provide cues or written words in margin as prompt	■ Refer to Appendix (A4)

Possible Classroom Problem	Possible Practical Approach	Further Advice via SENCO
Organizational skills (continued)		
■ Organizing work area/desk	■ Only essential items in work area – use a checklist Adult/peer support Encourage student to store work in appropriate folder, pocket file, etc. Consider using 'Work Schedules'	■ Refer to Occupational Therapy sheet (**OT7**) ■ Refer to Appendix (**A5**)
■ Use of ICT equipment	■ Diagrammatic step-by-step guide on how to set up equipment and cue cards for more specific tasks Ensure student e.g. is familiar with software Designated bag to carry equipment in with contents list Use labels to identify discs	■ Seek advice from school ICT department
■ Presentation and layout of written work	■ Cue sheet showing sample layout – concrete example, visual plan. Use part-prepared sheets Jot down essential points to be included, order and number them before writing in full format, crossing off jotting sheet Use 'writing frames' Fold paper or draw extra lines to reinforce awareness of columns Use lined/squared paper and pre-ruled margins	■ Refer to Further reading
■ Presentation and layout of drawn work, e.g. maps, tables, diagrams	■ Use part-prepared diagrams which need annotation Use stencils, templates Allow student to trace from text book Cue sheet showing sample layout – concrete example Fold paper or draw extra lines to e.g. aid positioning and awareness of columns, e.g. indentations for tables	

Table 3.6 History

Possible Classroom Problem	Possible Practical Approach	Further Advice via SENCO
Visual motor integration	**It may be necessary to seek advice from your SENCO in order to implement some of these approaches**	**Refer to visual motor integration skill sheet (F6)**
■ Accurate manipulative skills due to poor eye–hand co-ordination, e.g. model-making, scissors, rulers	■ Check posture and ensure stability with elbows resting on table Adult support when accuracy is paramount	■ Refer to Occupational Therapy sheet (**OT1**)
■ Accurate placement of component parts in relation to size, length, depth, height, orientation when drawing	■ Provide adult support to explore properties of finished product prior to drawing Discuss properties of component parts in relation to the whole	
■ Neatness and presentation of handwriting	■ Provide notes and worksheets, to reduce the amount of writing/copying Use bullet points rather than full sentence construction Use appropriate lined paper to help letters sit on the line Consider allowing longer time to complete task or adult support as a scribe Use alternative recording methods, e.g. dictaphone, appropriate ICT, part-prepared worksheets Consider extra time or adult support as a scribe in exam situations	■ Seek advice from ICT advisor, refer to Appendices (**A3** and **A1**) ■ Seek advice from educational psychologist
■ Producing illustrations to enhance written work	■ Use alternatives, e.g. Clip Art™, computer graphics, stencils Allow student to trace illustration from text book Adult support to produce illustrations	

Possible Classroom Problem

Possible Practical Approach

Further advice via SENCO

Possible Classroom Problem	Possible Practical Approach	Further advice via SENCO
Visual spatial relationships	**It may be necessary to seek advice from your SENCO in order to implement some of these approaches**	**Refer to visual spatial relationships skill sheet (F7)**
■ Uniformity e.g. of shape, size, spacing and slope of letters	■ Use squared/lined paper to help sizing and placing. Use prompt card for word spacing Encourage self-monitoring by using 'rules for writing tasks'	■ Refer to Occupational Therapy sheet (**OT3**)
■ Interpreting a range of layouts, e.g. pictures, aerial photographs, artefacts, photographs	■ Break down task and explain process in small steps Provide concrete examples to reinforce position in space, directional components, etc. Use computer software, e.g virtual reality	
■ Linear and vertical scanning	■ Reinforce working left to right, top to bottom and use of margin as a reference point Use clear perspex ruler as a line tracker, or for grids use two rulers positioned at 90° to one another Use squared paper to help with placing Colour code axis, tables, maps	■ Refer to Foundation skill sheet (**F5**), Appendix (**A4**)
■ Drawing maps, plans, artefacts representing information seen during field trips, museum visits	■ Talk through scale and position of objects/buildings Use squared paper to help with interpretation of scale and placing of features Encourage student to mark position of key objects on a pre-drawn grid during trip	
■ Drawing cross-sections of historical remains	■ Discuss relative positions of parts using a model	
■ Use of maps/plans on fieldwork trips, museum visits	■ Buddy working/adult support Ensure material is modified prior to field trip, e.g. highlight route, colour code axis	
■ Relating information seen on field trip to the whole, e.g. ruins of castle to scaled plan of castle	■ Discuss with an adult the relationships of the concrete form, e.g. castle with corresponding part on map/plan	

Table 3.6 History

Possible Classroom Problem	Possible Practical Approach	Further Advice via SENCO
visual figure ground discrimination	**It may be necessary to seek advice from your SENCO in order to implement some of these approaches**	**Refer to visual figure ground skill sheet (F9)**
■ Preparation for lesson in general	■ Ensure personal timetable is not too cluttered and that student can read it Limit amount of information on a page/board Limit amount of copying from board Reduce clutter on table or board Colour or highlight key information on page or board	■ Refer to Foundation skill sheet (**F5**) Appendix (**A4**)
■ Obtaining information from an atlas, plan, document, picture, photograph	■ Reinforce scanning left to right, top to bottom Use appropriate-sized windows to reduce visual field and highlight specific areas Use photocopier to enlarge material Highlight specific information on material	
■ Reading and interpreting information from information communications technology based sources, e.g. internet, computer printout	■ Use line trackers, appropriate-sized windows Colour code/highlight information Enlarge font size	■ Refer to Equipment resources (**ER**)
■ Selecting information from dictionary/indexes in reference book/multiple-choice sheets, etc.	■ Use line trackers, appropriate-sized windows to highlight specific areas Try coloured overlays Use dictionaries with alphabet tabs Use different colours when preparing multiple-choice questions	■ Refer to Equipment resources (**ER**)
■ Ability to e.g. partake in field trips, e.g. using maps, plans, museum signs	■ Use buddy working/adult supervision Ensure material is e.g. modified prior to field trip, e.g. enlarge material, use highlighters to indicate important information	■ Refer to Foundation skill sheet (**F5**) ■ Refer to Equipment resources (**ER**)
■ Seeing and recognizing artifacts on display in museums, galleries, etc.	■ Use buddy working/adult support Provide pictorial cue cards to match with artefacts	

Occupational Therapy Approaches for Secondary Special Needs © Whurr Publishers Ltd 2002

CA6 History (continued)

Possible Classroom Problem	Possible Practical Approach	Further Advice via SENCO
Visual form constancy	**It may be necessary to seek advice from your SENCO in order to implement some of these approaches**	**Refer to visual form constancy skill sheet (F8)**
■ Recognizing the same information in different formats, e.g. aerial photographs, satellite images	■ Use a model to demonstrate changes in orientation Provide adult/peer support to discuss properties of format and highlight key points on format	
■ Recognizing the same letter/word when presented in different handwriting styles, type face, font	■ Heighten staff awareness to student's difficulty Ensure work is presented in a consistent handwriting style, typeface, font where possible Provide peer/adult support	
Visual closure	**It may be necessary to seek advice from your SENCO in order to implement some of these approaches**	**Refer to visual closure skill sheet (F10)**
■ Fluency/speed of reading and spelling	■ Use a line tracker/clear ruler Limit the amount of information given Allow extra time to process information Reduce the amount of reading aloud in front of class if this is likely to have an effect in self-esteem Use spellchecker	■ Refer to Equipment resources (**ER**)
■ Relating information seen on field trip to the whole, e.g. ruins of castle to visual image of original castle	■ Discuss relationship of information gathered with an adult and relate to plan, picture, article	
■ Relating pieces of historical artifacts to the original article	■ Use concrete examples	■ Refer to Equipment resources (**ER**)
Visual memory/sequential memory	**It may be necessary to seek advice from your SENCO in order to implement some of these approaches**	**Refer to visual memory/sequential memory skill sheet (F11)**
■ Remembering historical information presented on a time line	■ Use alternative memory strategies, e.g. mnemonics, verbal/auditory skills	
■ Recalling chronological information about historical events	■ Make prompt card/cue sheet Use alternative memory strategies, e.g. auditory/verbal skills, mnemonics	

CA6 **History** (continued)

Possible Classroom Problem	Possible Practical Approach	Further advice via SENCO
Visual memory/visual sequential memory (continued)		
■ Copying information from board/book	■ Provide own desk top copy and place in optimum position for ease of scanning Use pre-prepared/part pre-prepared worksheets to reduce copying from board/book	■ Refer to Foundation skill sheet (**F5**)
■ Spelling historical vocabulary	■ Make a subject-specific word list	
■ Remembering landmarks on field trips	■ Encourage student to make notes, sketches, diagrams during trip Use numbered pictorial cue cards	
■ Making notes	■ Use adult support to check through notes Provide word bank of common mis-spelt words	
Auditory processing and memory	**It may be necessary to seek advice from your SENCO in order to implement some of these approaches**	**Refer to auditory processing and memory skill sheet (F12)**
■ Following and remembering verbal instructions/information	■ Use dictaphone Give clear, concise instructions in small steps Repeat instructions and allow student to verbalize back to check he or she has heard and understood Reinforce with written notes Withdraw student to quiet area and give assistance	■ Seek advice from speech and language therapist
■ Group discussion, e.g. ability to sift, summarize, cite evidence	■ Frequent resumé of essential points by group leader Encourage student to record main points of discussion and write down any questions during discussion Ask student leading questions as a prompt Use mind-mapping techniques Allow extra time for student to answer	■ Seek advice speech and language therapist
■ Participation in role play	■ Give small achievable parts. Encourage student to make own prompt sheet	■ Refer to Further reading
■ Listening and responding in discussions	■ Give advance warning of forthcoming discussion Check position in class, e.g. sitting in front/ facing speaker Use buddy working/adult support Use pre-prepared cue cards	

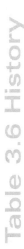

Possible Classroom Problem	Possible Practical Approach	Further Advice via SENCO
Social interaction	**It may be necessary to seek advice from your SENCO in order to implement some of these approaches**	**Refer to social interaction skill sheet (F13)**
■ Appropriate use of language, e.g. discussion/debate	■ Plan and initiate working groups with clear guidelines, e.g. debating rules	
■ Role play inability to assume role and react in character insufficient information to take on character role	■ Use discussion video, mime, to help develop spontaneous responses Cue cards Discuss role with partner/group members Allow extra time to practice	
■ Working as part of a group	■ Select group members carefully Allocate achievable task to student Adult facilitation	
■ Impulsiveness on field trips	■ Consider safety implications and undertake risk assessment Heighten teacher's and peers' awareness Select group members carefully	■ Refer to school field trips policy

CA7

Table 3.7 Geography

Possible Classroom Problem	Possible Practical Approach	Further advice via SENCO
Gross motor co-ordination	**It may be necessary to seek advice from your SENCO in order to implement some of these approaches**	**Refer to gross motor co-ordination skill sheet (F1)**
■ Ability to maintain functional writing posture	■ Check sitting position – chair/table size and height Consider working on an angled surface, e.g. clipboard, lever-arch file Provide rise and fall table with tilting surface	■ Refer to Occupational Therapy sheet (**OT1**), Equipment resources (**ER**) ■ Refer to Equipment resources (**ER**)
■ Reduced stamina for extended periods of writing Reduced quantity of written work which will include completion of homework	■ Alternative recording methods, e.g. dictaphone, appropriate ICT, voice-activated computer software, part-prepared notes and worksheets with spacing to reduce the amount of recording Consider adult support as an amanuensis Encouraging editing of work Bullet points rather than sentence construction, e.g. use 'writing frames' Give realistic targets – set attainable goals Allow student to re-establish posture by standing, stretching, etc. at agreed time intervals, i.e. 15 minutes Consider extending time to complete task Consider extra time allowance and fatigue breaks in exams Record homework using dictaphone/tape recorder for transcribing later Attend homework club (arranged by SENCO) if not too fatigued	■ Seek advice from ICT advisor, refer to Appendices (**A1** and **A3**) ■ Refer to Further reading ■ Seek advice from educational psychologist
■ Mobility around the classroom	■ Review position in class – consider sitting student end of row/table or near aisle Identify safe route by avoiding stepping over bags, feet Keep pathways clear	
■ Stamina and standing tolerance on field trips	■ Use fold-up shooting stick for rest periods Provide piece of waterproof fabric to sit on Choose group members carefully Allocate appropriate roles in group Undertake risk assessment	■ Refer to school field trip policy and school/health and safety representative/policy

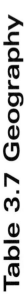

Occupational Therapy Approaches for Secondary Special Needs © Whurr Publishers Ltd 2002

CA7 Geography (continued)

Possible Classroom Problem	Possible Practical Approach	Further Advice via SENCO
Gross motor co-ordination (continued)		
■ Carrying equipment, e.g. in class, on field trips	■ Work in small groups and allocate specific equipment to each student Use a carrying aid, e.g trolley, backpack Undertake risk assessment	■ Refer to school manual handling policy/advisor
■ Participating in field trips, e.g. climbing stile, scrambling over rocks/stepping stones	■ Undertake risk assessment Consider safety implications Consider buddy working/adult support	■ Refer to school field trip policy and school/health and safety representative/policy
Fine motor dexterity	**It may be necessary to seek advice from your SENCO in order to implement some of these approaches**	**Refer to fine motor dexterity skill sheet (F2)**
■ Neatness and presentation of work	■ Check sitting posture-chair/table size and height Use lined paper to help with letter placement Consider adult support as a scribe (amanuensis) Consider alternative recording methods, e.g. dictaphone, appropriate ICT, part-prepared worksheets	■ Refer to Occupational Therapy sheet (**OT1**) ■ Seek advice from ICT advisor, refer to Appendices (**A1** and **A3**)
■ Fluency and speed of handwriting	■ Consider alternative pencil grasps and trial different writing tools Encourage pressure awareness and look at paper textures Consider working on an angled surface, e.g. clipboard, lever-arch file Consider alternative recording methods, e.g. dictaphone, appropriate ICT, part-prepared worksheets, adult support as an amanuensis	■ Refer to Occupational Therapy sheet (**OT1**), Equipment resources (**ER**), Appendix (**A2**) ■ Seek advice from ICT advisor, refer to Appendices (**A1** and **A3**)
■ Submitting incomplete homework	■ Record homework on dictaphone/tape recorder for transcribing later Provide part-prepared worksheets with spaces Consider student's difficulties when setting homework	

Table 3.7 Geography

Possible Classroom Problem	Possible Practical Approach	Further Advice via SENCO
Fine motor dexterity (continued)		
■ Using ICT equipment due to reduced keyboard and mouse skills	■ Consider providing adult help to set up and carry equipment from class to class Provide sufficient forearm support – use an appropriate-sized table and wrist rest/support Teach keyboard/touch typing skills to improve fluency Colour code keys on keyboard Try alternative mouse devices and keyboards Use 'dampening' facility to reduce repetition when key is depressed for too long Use a keyguard to improve accuracy	■ Refer to Equipment resources (**ER**) ■ Seek advice from ICT advisor, refer to Appendix (**A3**) ■ Refer to Equipment resources (**ER**)
■ Using instruments/equipment, e.g. ruler, scissors, compass	■ Trial alternative equipment Consider buddy working/adult support	■ Refer to Equipment resources (**ER**) and seek advice from occupational therapist, advisory teacher
■ Drawing accurate maps, diagrams, graphs	■ Use stencils, templates Allow student to trace diagram, etc. from text book Provide part-prepared worksheets which only need to be labelled Use appropriate ICT, e.g. computer graphics	■ Refer to Equipment resources (**ER**)
■ Model-making	■ Consider alternative materials, e.g. foam Use, velcro, pre-cut-out templates Consider buddy working/adult support	

Occupational Therapy Approaches for Secondary Special Needs © Whurr Publishers Ltd 2002

Possible Classroom Problem

Possible Practical Approach

Further Advice via SENCO

Organizational skills	It may be necessary to seek advice from your SENCO in order to implement some of these approaches	Refer to organizational skill sheet (F3)
■ Ability to follow verbal instructions	■ Reinforce with written notes on the board or e.g. on desk Give instructions in small steps and repeat Ask student to repeat instructions back to check they have heard and understood. If possible withdraw to quiet area and give assistance Give assistance to ensure homework instructions are understood	■ Seek advice from speech and language therapists
■ Ability to follow written instructions	■ Break instructions down into small steps Write instructions in point form, underline/highlight key instructions If possible, withdraw to quiet area and give assistance Consider buddy working/adult support	
■ Organizing thought process to express clearly cause and effect	■ Give prompts (verbal or written) Ask leading questions. Use mind-mapping techniques Allow student time to answer	■ Seek advice from educational psychologist ■ Refer to Further reading
■ Selecting appropriate information, e.g. from written text, maps	■ Give student cue card listing what to look for in text, map Use highlighters/colour coding systems Provide cues or write words in margin as a prompt Ensure directions and compass points are on maps	
■ Orientation of self and map in practical situations	■ Practise using compass on map Teach how to use fixed points of reference to oriente self	
■ Locating points of reference on a globe, atlas	■ Use of stickers, flags and colour-coded areas	

Table 3.7 Geography

Possible Classroom Problem	Possible Practical Approach	Further Advice via SENCO
Organizational skills (continued)		
■ Organizing work area/desk	■ Only essential items in work area – use checklists Encourage student to store work in appropriate folder, pocket file, etc. as they are working Consider using 'work schedules' Provide adult/peer support	■ Refer to Appendix (**A5**)
■ Using ICT equipment	■ Diagrammatic step-by-step guide on how to set up equipment and cue cards for more specific tasks Use labels to identify discs Ensure student is familiar with software Designated bag for carrying equipment with contents list	■ Seek advice from school ICT department
■ Presentation and layout of written work	■ Cue sheet showing sample layout – concrete example, visual plan Use part-prepared sheets Jot down essential points to be included, order them before writing in full format, crossing off jotting sheet Use of 'writing frames' Fold paper or draw extra lines to reinforce awareness of columns, e.g. indentations. Use lined/squared paper and pre-ruled margins Use appropriate ICT	■ Refer to Further reading ■ Seek advice from ICT advisor, refer to Appendix (**A3**)
■ Presentation and layout of drawn work, e.g. maps, graphs, diagrams	■ Use part-prepared diagrams ready for anotation Use stencils, templates Allow student to trace from text book Cue sheet showing sample layout Fold paper or draw extra lines to aid positioning	■ Refer to Equipment resources (**ER**)

Occupational Therapy Approaches for Secondary Special Needs © Whurr Publishers Ltd 2002

CA7 Geography (continued)

Possible Classroom Problem | Possible Practical Approach | Further Advice via SENCO

Possible Classroom Problem	Possible Practical Approach	Further Advice via SENCO
Visual motor integration	**It may be necessary to seek advice from your SENCO in order to implement some of these approaches**	**Refer to visual motor integration skill sheet (F6)**
■ Presentation of handwriting	■ Provide notes and worksheets to reduce the amount of recording Use bullet points rather than full sentence construction Use appropriate lined paper to help letters sit on the line Consider allowing longer time to complete task Consider extra time allowance in exams/adult support as an amanuensts Use alternative recording methods, e.g. dictaphone, word processor, adult support as an amanuensts	■ Seek advice from educational psychologist
■ Accuracy of manipulative skills due to poor eye–hand co-ordination, e.g. model-making, scissors, rulers, compass, scale rule	■ Check posture to ensure optimum stability with elbows resting on tables Undertake risk assessment Provide adult support when accuracy is paramount and when there are safety implications	■ Refer to Occupational Therapy sheet (**OT1**) ■ Seek advice from school health and safety representative
■ Ability to use perspective for drawing	■ Explore properties of finished product prior to drawing Discuss properties of component parts in relation to whole	
■ Accurate placement of component parts in relation to size, length, depth, height orientation when drawing	■ Explore properties of finished product prior to drawing Discuss properties of component parts in relationship to the whole	
■ Producing illustrations to enhance written work	■ Use alternatives, e.g. Clip Art™, computer graphics, stencils, pre-drawn work which only needs to be labelled Adult support to produce illustrations Allow student to trace illustration from text book	■ Seek advice from ICT advisor, refer to Equipment resources (**ER**)

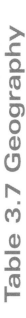

CA7

Table 3.7 Geography

Possible Classroom Problem	Possible Practical Approach	Further Advice via SENCO
Visual spatial relationships	**It may be necessary to seek advice from your SENCO** **In order to implement some of these approaches**	**Refer to visual spatial relationships** **skill sheet (F7)**
■ Uniformity of shape, size, spacing and slope of letters	■ Use squared/lined paper to help size and placement. Use prompt card for word spacing Encourage self-monitoring by using 'rules for writing tasks'	■ Refer to Appendix (**A2**) ■ Refer to Occupational Therapy sheet (**OT3**)
■ Interpreting a range of layouts, e.g. maps, graphs, satellite images, aerial photographs	■ Reinforce compass points and directional components Break down task and explain process in small steps Provide concrete examples to reinforce position in space, directional components, etc. Use computer software, e.g. virtual reality	
■ Linear and vertical scanning	■ Reinforce working left to right, top to bottom and use margin as a reference point Use clear perspex ruler as a line tracker or for grids use two rulers positioned at 90° to one another Use squared paper to help with placing Colour code axis on graphs, tables, maps	■ Refer to Foundation skill sheet (**F5**) and Appendix (**A4**)
■ Drawing maps and plans using a variety of scales	■ Use squared paper to help with interpretation of scale and placement of features Talk through scale using concrete examples, e.g. scale rulers Use stencil/templates and appropriate ICT software	■ Refer to Equipment resources (**ER**)
■ Drawing maps or plans representing information seen during field trips, e.g. of a town or countryside	■ Use squared/graph paper to help with interpretation of scale and placement of features Talk through scale and position of objects/buildings Use stencils, templates Encourage student to mark position of key landmarks on a pre-drawn grid during the field trip	■ Refer to Equipment resources (**ER**)
■ Relating information seen on field trips to the whole, e.g. ruins of castle to scale plan of castle	■ Discuss with an adult the relationship of the concrete form with corresponding part on plan	

Occupational Therapy Approaches for Secondary Special Needs © Whurr Publishers Ltd 2002

CA7 **Geography** (continued)

Possible Classroom Problem	Possible Practical Approach	Further Advice via SENCO
Visual spatial relationships (continued)		
■ Drawing cross-sections of geological forms	■ Discuss relative positions of component part using a model	
■ Understanding and interpreting relative scale, distances, size on maps, drawings	■ Ensure student has fully understood the concept of scale Reinforce the teaching of perspectives	
■ Use of maps on field work trips	■ Buddy working/adult support Ensure material is modified prior to field trip, e.g. highlight route or colour code axis	
■ Identifying relief and landscape features on OS map	■ Use cue card or acetate with contour lines Work with a buddy who has a clear understanding	
Visual figure ground discrimination	**It may be necessary to seek advice from your SENCO in order to implement some of these approaches**	**Refer to visual figure ground skill sheet (F9)**
■ Preparation for lesson in general	■ Ensure personal timetable is not too cluttered and that student can read it Limit amount of information on a page/board Limit amount of copying from board Reduce clutter on table or board Colour or highlight key information on page or board	
■ Selecting information to find grid references	■ Colour code axis Use line trackers, appropriate-sized windows to highlight specific areas Try coloured overlays	■ Refer to Equipment resources (**ER**) ■ Refer to Foundation skill sheet (**F5**)
■ Finding specific place or obtaining information from a map, globe, atlas, plans, satellite images, graphs/tables	■ Reinforce scanning left to right, top to bottom Use appropriate-sized windows to reduce visual field Use map plan with larger scale or enlarge original Use photocopier to enlarge material Colour code axis/highlight specific information on graph, table Use a laminated map symbol strip	■ Refer to Foundation skill sheet (**F5**) and Appendix (**A4**)

Occupational Therapy Approaches for Secondary Special Needs © Whurr Publishers Ltd 2002

Table 3.7 Geography

Possible Classroom Problem	Possible Practical Approach	Further Advice via SENCO
Visual figure ground discrimination (continued)		
Finding relevant symbol, key and scale in the symbol guide and on a map, etc.	Highlight/mark relevant symbol on laminated symbol strip with a washable pen Use appropriate-sized window in a left to right, top to bottom sequence to highlight specific area	Refer to Equipment resources (**ER**)
Reading and interpreting information from ICT-based sources, e.g. internet, computer printout, satellite images, mapping software	Use line trackers, appropriate-sized windows Colour code/highlight information Enlarge font size	
Ability to partake in field trips, e.g. using maps, plans, road signs	Use buddy working/adult support Ensure material is modified prior to field trip, e.g. enlarge material, use highlighters to indicate important information	
Visual form constancy	**It may be necessary to seek advice from SENCO in order to implement some of these approaches**	**Refer to visual form constancy skill sheet (F8)**
Recognizing country outlines regardless of size, scale, colour	Use multi-sensory and ICT approaches to learning Reinforce common properties of outline Draw country on acetate to match with outline on map	
Understanding the relationship between different scales	Give detailed explanation of properties of scale	
Recognizing the same information in different formats, e.g. aerial photographs, satellite images	Use a model to demonstrate changes in orientation Provide adult/peer support to discuss properties of photographs/images and highlight key points on image, maps, photographs	

164

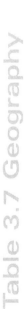

Possible Classroom Problem	Possible Practical Approach	Further Advice via SENCO
visual closure	**It may be necessary to seek advice from your SENCO in order to implement some of these approaches**	**Refer to visual closure skill sheet (F10)**
■ Fluency/speed of reading and spelling	■ Use a line tracker/clear ruler as a visual guide Limit the amount of information given Allow extra time to process information Reduce the amount of reading aloud in front of class if this is likely to have an effect on self-esteem Use spellchecker	■ Refer to Equipment resources (**ER**)
■ Relating information seen on field trips to the whole, e.g. geological strata	■ Discuss relationship of information gathered with adult and relate to diagram, map	■ Refer to Equipment resources (**ER**)
■ Relating geomorphological, e.g. erosions and their effects on people and landscapes	■ Consider adult support to reinforce process	
■ Relating part of map to the whole map	■ Provide picture/map of complete area and highlight part/section	
■ Understanding cyclical processing, e.g. water stages, ecosystem	■ Use prompt cards to identify each stage of cycle and talk through process	
visual memory/sequential memory	**It may be necessary to seek advice from your SENCO in order to implement some of these approaches**	**Refer to visual memory/sequential memory skill sheet (F11)**
■ Remembering grid/map references	■ Encourage student to write out grid reference onto map/note pad	
■ Recalling statistical information about countries	■ Make prompt card/cue sheet Use alternative memory strategies, e.g. auditory skills, verbal skills, mnemonics	
■ Copying information from board/book	■ Provide own desktop copy and place in optimum position for ease of scanning Use pre-prepared/part-prepared worksheets to reduce copying from board/book	■ Refer to Foundation skill sheet (**F5**), Appendix (**A4**)
■ Spelling geographical vocabulary	■ Make a subject specific vocabulary list	

Table 3.7 Geography

Possible Classroom Problem	Possible Practical Approach	Further Advice via SENCO
visual memory/sequential memory (continued)		
Remembering symbols/keys on maps	■ Make a cue card of commonly used symbols Reinforce pictorial representation with auditory description	
Remembering common shapes, e.g. outline of counties/continents	■ Awareness that student may need extra time to learn shape Try using multi-sensory and ICT approaches to learning Draw country/continents on acetate and match with outline on map	
Remembering landmarks on field trips	■ Encourage student to make notes/sketches/diagrams during the trip Use numbered pictorial cue card Use headings of a memory cue	
Making notes	■ Use adult support to check through notes Provide word bank of common misspelt words	
Auditory processing and memory	**It may be necessary to seek advice from your SENCO in order to implement some of these approaches**	**Refer to auditory processing and memory skill sheet (F12)**
Listening and remembering information, e.g. grid references	■ Give clear concise instructions and repeat if necessary Reinforce written notes Write information on the board Provide student with written grid references Get student to record own references before starting task	■ Seek advice from speech and language therapist
Understanding geographical terminology	■ Use subject specific vocabulary lists	
Following and remembering instructions/information	■ Use dictaphone Give clear, concise instructions and allow student to verbalize back to check they have heard and understood Reinforce with written notes Consider use of 'work schedules'	■ Refer to Appendix (A5)

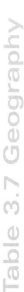

166

Occupational Therapy Approaches for Secondary Special Needs © Whurr Publishers Ltd 2002

CA7 Geography (continued)

Possible Classroom Problem	Possible Practical Approach	Further Advice via SENCO
Auditory memory and processing (continued)		
■ Group discussion, e.g. ability to sift and summarize, use salient points, cite evidence	■ Frequent resumé of essential points by group leader Encourage student to record main points of discussion and write down any questions during discussion Ask student leading questions as a prompt Use mind-mapping techniques Allow time for student to answer	■ Refer to Further reading
Social interaction	**It may be necessary to seek advice from your SENCO in order to implement some of these approaches**	**Refer to social interaction skill sheet (F13)**
■ Group discussion	■ Give advance warning of forthcoming discussion Check position in class, e.g. sitting in front or facing speaker Use mind-mapping techniques Allow extra time for student to answer Use buddy working/adult support Use pre-prepared cue cards	■ Refer to Further reading
■ Working as part of a group on field trips	■ Select group members carefully Allocate achievable task to student Adult facilitation	
■ Impulsiveness on field trips	■ Consider safety implications and undertake risk assessment Heighten teacher's and peers' awareness Select group members carefully	■ Refer to school trips policy and guidelines

CA8

Table 3.8 Modern foreign languages

Possible Classroom Problem	Possible Practical Approach	Further Advice via SENCO
Gross motor co-ordination	**It may be necessary to seek advice from your SENCO in order to implement some of these approaches**	**Refer to gross motor skill sheet (F1)**
■ Ability to maintain functional writing posture	■ Check sitting posture – chair/table size and height Consider working on angled surface, e.g. clipboard, lever-arch file Provide rise and fall table with tilting surface	■ Refer to Occupational Therapy sheet (**OT1**), Equipment resources (**ER**) ■ Refer to Equipment resources (**ER**)
■ Reduced stamina for e.g. extended periods of writing Reduced quantity of written work which will include completion of homework	■ Alternative recording methods, e.g. appropriate ICT, voice-activated computer software, dictaphone, part-prepared worksheets with spacing to be filled in Consider adult support as an amanuensts Encourage editing of work Bullet points rather than full sentence construction, e.g. use 'writing frames' Give realistic targets – set individual attainable goals Consider extending time to complete task Consider extra time allowance and fatigue breaks in exams Allow student to re-establish posture by standing, stretching, etc. at agreed time intervals, e.g. 15 minutes	■ Seek advice from ICT advisor and refer to Appendices (**A1** and **A3**) ■ Refer to Further reading ■ Seek advice from educational psychologist
Fine motor dexterity	**It may be necessary to seek advice from your SENCO in order to implement some of these approaches**	**Refer to fine motor dexterity skill sheet (F2)**
■ Neatness of handwriting and presentation of work Fluency and speed of handwriting	■ Check sitting posture – chair/table size and height Consider working on an angled surface, e.g. clipboard, lever-arch file Consider alternative pencil grasps and trial different writing tools Use appropriate lined paper to help with letter placement Accept that quantity of written work will be reduced Consider adult support as an anenuensis	■ Refer to Occupational Therapy sheet (**OT1**) and Equipment resources (**ER**)
	■ Consider alternative recording methods, e.g. dictaphone, appropriate ICT, part-prepared worksheets with spaces to be filled in Consider extra time allowance or adult support as an amanuensts in exam situations	■ Seek advice from ICT advisor and refer to Appendices (**A3** and **A1**) ■ Seek advice from educational psychologist
■ Use of audio recording material	■ Consider using alternative equipment Consider buddy working/adult support	

CA8 Modern foreign languages (continued)

Occupational Therapy Approaches for Secondary Special Needs © Whurr Publishers Ltd 2002

Possible Classroom Problem	Possible Practical Approach	Further Advice via SENCO
Organizational skills	**It may be necessary to seek advice from your SENCO in order to implement some of these approaches**	**Refer to organizational skill sheet (F3)**
■ Preparation for school day and subject	■ Additional training to use school organizer/homework diary Use a daily timetable with each subject identified by a different coloured dot Colour code books to correspond with subjects, e.g. French blue, Spanish green, English red (use coloured plastic exercise book covers) List books/items needed for each subject	■ Refer to Occupational Therapy sheet (**OT7**)
■ Presentation and layout of written work/tables	■ Cue sheet showing sample layout – concrete example, visual plan Use part-prepared sheets with spaces to be filled in Jot down essential points to be included, order and number them before writing in final form Use 'writing frames' and mind-mapping techniques Fold paper or draw extra lines to reinforce awareness of columns, e.g. verb tables Use lined/squared paper	■ Refer to Further reading
■ Organizing work area/desk	■ Only essential items in work area – use a checklist Adult/peer support Consider position in class, e.g. place student so left- and right-handed students are not colliding	
■ Using ICT equipment for accessing and communicating information	■ Provide diagrammatic step-by-step guide/cue cards on how to set up and use the equipment Ensure student is familiar with software/equipment	■ Seek advice from school ICT department
■ Ability to follow verbal instructions	■ Reinforce with written/pictorial notes Give instructions in small steps and repeat instructions as necessary Ask student to repeat instructions back to check they have heard and understood If possible withdraw to quiet area and give assistance Provide assistance to ensure homework instructions are understood – use a homework diary	■ Seek advice from speech and language therapist

CA8 Modern foreign languages (continued)

Occupational Therapy Approaches for Secondary Special Needs © Whurr Publishers Ltd 2002

Table 3.8 Modern foreign languages

Possible Classroom Problem	Possible Practical Approach	Further Advice via SENCO
Organizational skills (continued)		
■ Ability to follow written instructions	■ Break instructions down into small steps Write instructions in point form, underline/highlight key instructions	
■ Using indexes/dictionaries	■ Provide alphabet strip-stick on ruler or keep in pencil case Colour code alphabet strip, e.g. abc-red, def-blue Use dictionaries with tabs and clear, bold print on top of each page Use computer-based dictionaries with a search facility, e.g. Collins Oxford CD (French), Duden (German) and permanently install on network if possible	
■ Expressive skills, e.g. how to ask and answer questions, express opinions and identify feelings	■ Give verbal/written prompts Ask leading questions Use mind-mapping techniques Allow time for student to answer	■ Refer to Further reading
■ Selecting appropriate information from written text	■ Give student cue card listing information to look for in text Use highlighters/colour coding systems Provide cues or write words in margin as a prompt Use line tracker, appropriate-sized window card, clear ruler to highlight specific areas	■ Refer to Equipment resources (**ER**)
■ Summarizing and reporting key points of spoken language or written text	■ Highlight key points in written text. Encourage student to list key points of spoken text Extend use of audio equipment, dictaphone, etc.	
Visual motor integration	**It may be necessary to seek advice from your SENCO in order to implement some of these approaches**	**Refer to visual motor integration skill sheet (F6)**
■ Neatness and presentation of handwriting	■ Use alternative recording methods, e.g. dictaphone, appropriate ICT, pre-prepared worksheets with spaces for student to fill in Use appropriate lined paper to help with letter placement Consider allowing longer time to complete task Consider extra time allowance and adult support as an amamuensts in exam situations	■ Seek advice from ICT advisor and refer to Appendices (**A1** and **A3**) ■ Seek advice with educational psychologist

Occupational Therapy Approaches for Secondary Special Needs © Whurr Publishers Ltd 2002

CA8 Modern foreign languages (continued)

Possible Classroom Problem	Possible Practical Approach	Further Advice via SENCO
Visual motor integration (continued)		
■ Producing illustrations to enhance written work	■ Use Clip Art™, computer graphics Use stickers/stencils Allow student to trace illustrations from text books	
Visual spatial relationships	**It may be necessary to seek advice from your SENCO in order to implement some of these approaches**	**Refer to visual spatial relationships skill sheet (F7)**
■ Uniformity of shape, size, spacing, slope of letters and accents	■ Use squared/lined paper to help sizing and placement Use prompt card for word spacing and position of accents Encourage self-monitoring by using 'rules for writing tasks'	■ Refer to Occupational Therapy sheet (**OT3**), Appendix (**A2**)
■ Producing work in a range of formats, e.g. newspapers, posters	■ Give concrete example of expected format Prepared templates in various shapes and size to help arrange layout before transferring to paper Use part-prepared layout	
■ Linear and vertical scanning	■ Reinforce working left to right, top to bottom and use of margin as a reference point Use clear perspex ruler as a line tracker Produce work on squared paper	■ Refer to Foundation skill sheet (**F5**), Appendix (**A4**)
visual figure ground discrimination	**It may be necessary to seek advice from your SENCO in order to implement some of these approaches**	**Refer to visual figure ground skill sheet (F9)**
■ Preparation for lesson in general	■ Limit amount of information on a page/board Reduce clutter on table or board Colour or highlight key information on page or board	■ Refer to Occupational Therapy sheet (**OT7**)
■ Selecting information from a multiple-choice sheet, dictionary, indexes	■ Use a line tracker/appropriate sized windows to highlight specific areas Pre-prepare dictionary by highlighting first letter of each word Use a dictionary which is clearly laid out Provide computer-based dictionaries with search facility, e.g. Collins Oxford CD (French), Duden (German) and permanently install on network if possible	■ Refer to Equipment resources (**ER**), Appendix (**A4**)

CA8 Modern foreign languages (continued)

Table 3.8 Modern foreign languages

Possible Classroom Problem	Possible Practical Approach	Further Advice via SENCO
Visual figure ground discrimination (continued)		
■ Selecting information from a multiple-choice sheet, dictionary, indexes (continued)	Alternate different colours when preparing multiple-choice questions	
■ Finding place in a range of layouts, e.g. text, newspapers, books, email, Internet screen	Reinforce scanning left to right, top to bottom Consider using different formats to highlight key points, e.g. fonts, type face, blocking, bullet points, bold Underline or highlight each new section Use a line tracker/appropriate-sized window to highlight specific areas	■ Refer to Foundation skill sheet (**F5**) ■ Refer to Equipment resources (**ER**)
■ Proof reading and editing	Use pre-prepared cue card listing words that are consistently difficult for student to spell Use a line tracker to help with scanning	■ Refer to Equipment resources (**ER**)
Visual form constancy	**It may be necessary to seek advice from your SENCO in order to implement some of these approaches**	**Refer to visual form constancy skill sheet (F8)**
■ Difficulty developing a fluent handwriting script	■ Heighten awareness of student's problem ■ Use alternative methods of recording, e.g. appropriate ICT, adult support as an amanuensts, pre-prepared work sheets with spaces for student to fill in	■ Refer to Appendices (**A1** and **A3**) and Occupational Therapy sheet (**OT3**)
■ Recognizing the same letter/word when presented in different handwriting styles, type face, font	■ Heighten staff awareness ■ Consider peer/adult support Ensure work is presented in a consistent style, type face, font	
Visual closure	**It may be necessary to seek advice from your SENCO in order to implement some of these approaches**	**Refer to visual closure skill sheet (F10)**
■ Fluency/speed for reading and spelling	■ Check frequently whether content is understood Limit the amount of information given Use a line tracker/clear ruler to help with scanning Allow more time to process information Reduce amount of reading aloud in front of class because of potential effect on self-esteem Use teaching techniques which focus on auditory input	■ Refer to Foundation skill sheet (**F5**) ■ Refer to Equipment resources (**ER**)

CA8 Modern foreign languages (continued)

Possible Classroom Problem	Possible Practical Approach	Further Advice via SENCO
Visual memory/sequential memory	**It may be necessary to seek advice from your SENCO in order to implement some of these approaches**	**Refer to visual memory/sequential memory skill sheet (F11)**
■ Spelling	■ Use a dictionary which is clearly laid out and easy to read Provide an alphabet strip – placed on ruler, in pencil case Provide a list of commonly used words Practice recognition of visual patterns through games, e.g. shape blocks Break down difficult words into patterns thus enabling students to learn through visual sequences Use hand-held spell checker or computer software with in-built spell checker	■ Refer to Equipment resources (**ER**)
■ Remembering grammatical rules	■ Develop mnemonic strategies Use cue cards Practice rules – try highlighting endings Use phrase-based learning of commonly used grammatical construction	
■ Copying information from board	■ Reduce copying from board, e.g. use pre-prepared worksheets or give own copy of board information Be aware of objects, in line of vision, which could interfere with student's view Use different colours to differentiate sections of text to be copied Use stickers on board as visual markers Give adequate time for student to record work	■ Refer to Foundation skill sheet (**F5**), Appendix (**A4**)
■ Copying information from book/paper	■ Reduce copying from book, e.g. use pre-prepared worksheets Adult support to differentiate sections of text to be copied with coloured markers Explore optimum position of book/paper for ease of scanning	■ Refer to Foundation skill sheet (**F5**), Appendix (**A4**)
■ Making notes	■ Use adult support to check through notes Provide word bank of common misspelt words	

CA8 Modern foreign languages (continued)

Table 3.8 Modern foreign languages

Possible Classroom Problem	Possible Practical Approach	Further Advice via SENCO
Auditory processing and memory	**It may be necessary to seek advice from your SENCO in order to implement some of these approaches**	**Refer to auditory processing and memory skill sheet (F12)**
■ Remembering verbal instructions	■ Use dictaphone Give clear, concise instructions in small steps Repeat instructions and allow student to verbalize back in English to check that they have understood Reinforce with written notes in target language and English If possible withdraw student to quiet area and give assistance	■ Seek advice from speech and language therapist
■ Discriminating and processing auditory information	■ Reduce speed of delivery/pause between phrases and emphasize intonation Emphasis on phonetic structures Provide opportunity to listen to variations in accent/dialect	
■ Communicating in target language	■ Ensure role model uses correct pronunciation, especially where group work is involved Check position in class, e.g. sitting in front or facing speaker Give advance warning of forthcoming discussion Encourage student to record main points Ask student leading questions as a prompt Allow time for student to answer Frequent resumé of essential points	
Social interaction	**It may be necessary to seek advice from your SENCO in order to implement some of these approaches**	**Refer to social interaction skill sheet (F13)**
■ Differentiating target language to suit context, audience and purpose	■ Use role play Reinforce rules by using cue cards	
■ Assuming roles in practical sessions	■ Use video, mime and role play to help develop responses	
■ Low self-esteem leading to withdrawal	■ Heighten awareness of difficulties	
■ Working as part of a group	■ Select group members carefully Allocate achievable task Adult facilitation	

CA 8 Modern foreign languages

CA9

Table 3.9 Art

Possible Classroom Problem	Possible Practical Approach	Further Advice via SENCO
Gross motor co-ordination	**It may be necessary to seek advice from your SENCO in order to implement some of these approaches**	**Refer to gross motor skill sheet (F1)**
■ Ability to maintain functional working position in		■ Refer to Occupational Therapy sheet (**OT1**)
(a) sitting on high stool without back/foot support	■ Check sitting posture – stool/table size, height and angle Ensure adequate clearance for knees under table and support for forearms Consider use of rise and fall table Rest feet on crossbar of stool for support Consider stool with back – arrange for REMAP department to alter existing stools or buy alternative stool Set attainable goals as output may be reduced Consider working on an angled writing surface, e.g. clipboard, easel, table with an angled work surface Allow student to re-establish posture by standing, stretching at agreed time intervals.	■ Refer to Equipment resources (**ER**) ■ Refer to Equipment resources (**ER**), Useful addresses ■ Refer to Equipment resources (**ER**)
(b) standing	■ Check table/bench height relative to student Supply wooden platform if required, painted clearly for safety, e.g. bright yellow Consider providing benches/work surfaces which are height adjustable Ensure equipment for practical work is within reach Consider allowing student to sit for part of practical work Provide adequate areas to 'prop'	■ Refer to Occupational Therapy sheet (**OT1**) ■ Refer to workshop health and safety regulations ■ Refer to Equipment resources (**ER**) ■ Refer to workshop health and safety regulations
■ Reduced stamina for extended periods of painting, drawing, cutting	■ Ensure optimum supported working position is assumed, e.g. standing at an appropriate height work surface, support for forearms, use of angled surface Give realistic targets; set appropriate task Consider longer time to complete task Plan lesson so that heavy physical work is undertaken early in lesson or intersperse practical 'making' with 'designing' and recording	■ Refer to Occupational Therapy sheet (**OT1**), Equipment resources (**ER**)

Table 3.9 Art

Possible Classroom Problem	Possible Practical Approach	Further Advice via SENCO
Gross motor co-ordination (continued)		
■ Body awareness in practical group work	■ Undertake risk assessment Ensure there is adequate space to allow for uncoordinated movements Smaller groups for practical work Consider safety issues, raise student's awareness of the need to plan task methodically Consider the need for adult support	■ Seek advice from school health and safety representative/policy
■ Mobility around the classroom/workshop	■ Heighten awareness of the need to maintain uncluttered aisles Reduce the number of students moving around the art room at any one time – enforce clear rules 'for the room' Reduce student's need to move around the art room by collecting equipment before starting task Provide individual set of equipment Use temporary storage area for equipment, e.g. in centre of table to reduce risk of being knocked off	
■ Carrying materials and equipment	■ Undertake risk assessment Analyse work area for safe and efficient use of equipment Buddy working/adult support to carry equipment Consider alternative means of carrying/moving equipment, e.g. use plastic basket Observe correct lifting procedures	■ Seek advice from school health and safety representative ■ Refer to school manual handling policy
■ Handling/stabilizing large materials and equipment Setting up equipment	■ Undertake risk assessment Prioritize relevance of curricular task for student Observe safety rules, e.g. use cutting mats, protective clothing Consider stabilizing equipment, e.g. dycem mat, clamp Use smaller quantity of material, e.g. clay	■ Seek advice from school health and safety representative ■ Refer to Equipment resources (**ER**)
■ Grading force of movement	■ Seek alternative media – choose materials with appropriate density/resistance (refer to curricular requirements) Adult support/buddy working	

Occupational Therapy Approaches for Secondary Special Needs © Whurr Publishers Ltd 2002

CA9 Art (continued)

Possible Classroom Problem	Possible Practical Approach	Further Advice via SENCO
Gross motor co-ordination (continued)		
■ Access to and mobility around art gallery/museums	■ Pre-plan visit to gain accurate knowledge of area and facilities Consider safety implications – undertake risk assessment	■ Refer to school trips policy
■ Uncontrolled and imprecise movements leading to safety implications	■ Undertake risk assessment Consider safety issues, raise student's awareness of the need to plan task methodically Ensure only relevant materials/equipment on work surface Ensure there is adequate space to allow for uncontrolled movements Smaller groups for practical work Consider the need for adult support	■ Seek advice from school health and safety representative, refer to health and safety policy
■ Large construction tasks, e.g. collage/sculpture	■ Buddy working/adult support Plan lesson so that large tasks/physical work is undertaken early in lesson or intersperse practical 'making' with 'designing' and recording Select appropriate task for student's ability, enabling contribution to group task	
Fine motor dexterity	**It may be necessary to seek advice from your SENCO in order to implement some of these approaches**	**Refer to fine motor dexterity skill sheet (F2)**
■ Reduced safety resulting from poorly controlled or impulsive movements	■ Undertake risk assessment Raise awareness of safety issues resulting from poor manual dexterity Prioritize relevance of curricular task for student Consider providing adult support Analyse work area to ensure safe use of equipment, e.g ensure work space is uncluttered	■ Seek advice from school health and safety representative and refer to school health and safety policy.
■ Handling and manipulating equipment, e.g. scissors, stanley knives, aerosols, spray guns	■ Ensure good lighting Consider stabilizing equipment, e.g. with dycem mat, clamp Provide individual set of adapted equipment Trial alternative equipment, e.g. enlarged handles	■ Refer to Equipment resources (**ER**) ■ Seek advice from occupational therapist, advisory teacher

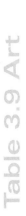

Possible Classroom Problem	Possible Practical Approach	Further Advice via SENCO
Fine motor dexterity (continued)		
■ Handling and manipulating equipment, e.g. scissors, stanley knives, aerosols, spray guns (continued)	■ Provide part prepared work to minimize necessity for fine precision movements Motor programme to improve strength/dexterity Consider adult support/buddy working	■ Refer to Occupational Therapy sheet (**OT5**)
■ Handling and measuring materials, e.g. solids, liquids, due to poor fine motor control and reduced ability to grade pressure of movement	■ Work with partner or adult when accuracy is paramount Seek alternative medium – choose tasks and materials with appropriate density/resistance (refer to curricular requirements) Use alternative measuring equipment which allows for imprecise movements	
■ Reduced tactile awareness, further impaired by wearing gloves	■ Encourage tactile awareness through a variety of textures, consistencies, surfaces, shape Ensure gloves are the correct size	
■ Grading of force for precise movements	■ Trial variety of media, e.g. chalk, pastels, ink, pen	
■ Ability to refine techniques	■ Work on a larger scale Heighten awareness of student's ability/limitations Set attainable tasks/goals Seek alternative outcomes, e.g. abstract techniques	
■ Neatness and presentation of work Fluency and speed of handwriting	■ Check working posture Use of appropriate lined/squared paper to help placement of work Consider alternative writing tools Accept the quantity of written work will be reduced Consider working on an angled surface, e.g. clipboard, lever-arch file, easel Consider alternative recording methods, e.g. dictaphone, appropriate ICT, adult support as an amanuensis, part-prepared worksheet Consider extra time allowance in exams or adult to act as amanuensis	■ Refer to Occupational Therapy sheets (**OT1**) ■ Refer to Equipment resources (**ER**) ■ Refer to Equipment resources (**ER**) ■ Seek advice from ICT advisor, refer to Appendices (**A1** and **A3**) ■ Seek advice from educational pyschologist

Possible Classroom Problem	Possible Practical Approach	Further Advice via SENCO
Fine motor dexterity (continued)		
■ Following health and safety procedures, e.g. putting on protective clothing/goggles/masks	■ Adapt fastenings, e.g. use velcro Use larger protective clothing which may be easier to put on Consider adult support/buddy working	■ Seek advice from occupational therapist
■ Using ICT equipment due to reduced keyboard and mouse skills	■ Provide sufficient forearm support, e.g. use appropriate sized table, wrist rest/support Trial alternative mouse devices and keyboards Use a keyguard to improve accuracy	■ Refer to Equipment resources (**ER**) Appendix (**A3**) ■ Seek advice from ICT advisor ■ Refer to Equipment resources (**ER**)
Organizational skills	**It may be necessary to seek advice from your SENCO in order to implement some of these approaches**	**Refer to organizational skill sheet (F3)**
■ Exploring and developing ideas	■ Create secure environment to encourage self-expression Use mind-mapping techniques Consider adult support	■ Refer to Further reading
■ Reduced health and safety awareness	■ Undertake risk assessments Use of safety checklists Encourage student to pre-plan task, planning far enough ahead to anticipate problems Adult input may be needed to help with problem or to steer student towards an easier route Consider buddy working/adult support Ensure work area is uncluttered	■ Seek advice from school health and safety representative and refer to school health and safety policy
■ Organizing design process and performing practical tasks	■ Plan stages of task prior to start Use mind-mapping techniques Use of checklists Consider use of 'work schedules' Consider 1:1 instruction on use of specific equipment, e.g. stanley knife Encourage rough sketches to help formulate ideas Give prompts and provide practical concrete example Use of part-prepared materials/media Refer to art resource materials for ideas	■ Refer to Further reading ■ Refer to Appendix (**A5**)

CA9 Art (continued)

Table 3.9 Art

Possible Classroom Problem	Possible Practical Approach	Further Advice via SENCO
Organizational skills (continued)		
■ Ability to follow verbal instructions	■ Reinforce with diagrammatic/written notes/pictorial cue cards Give instructions in small steps and repeat instructions frequently to ensure student has understood Provide frequent recapping – 'what we have done', 'what we will do next' Consider use of 'work schedules'	■ Seek advice from speech and language therapist ■ Refer to Appendix (**A5**)
■ Ability to follow written methodology	■ Break down written instructions into small steps, highlighting key points with highlighter pen Provide combined written and diagrammatic instructions Provide clear written methodology for art work	
■ Presentation and layout of written work and artistic forms	■ Use of alternative recording methods, e.g. part-prepared worksheets, stencils, appropriate ICT Give cue sheet with sample layout Use 'writing frames' Use of squared/graph/tracing paper Give concrete examples of expected positioning and layout Parallel working or adult support	■ Seek advice from ICT advisor ■ Refer to Further reading
■ Collating and storing art work	■ Use appropriate filing system, e.g. portfolio, art folder	
■ Negotiating self around art area to collect equipment or seek help	■ Ensure aisles are uncluttered Adequate pre-planning e.g. to ensure student has necessary equipment before starting Provide individual set of equipment Position tables/benches to allow for safe movement of individuals One group at a time to collect Heighten adult awareness to reduce need for student to leave task Check student's progress regularly	

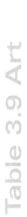

CA9 Art (continued)

Possible Classroom Problem	Possible Practical Approach	Further Advice via SENCO
visual motor integration	**It may be necessary to seek advice from your SENCO in order to implement some of these approaches**	**Refer to visual motor integration skill sheet (F6)**
■ Inaccurate manipulative skills due to poor eye – hand coordination, e.g. modelling tools, paintbrush, scissors	■ Choose activity carefully to enhance student's ability to succeed – consider relevance of curricular task Check posture and ensure stability with elbows resting on bench/table, although this may not be possible when using some equipment Consider adult support when accuracy is paramount	■ Seek advice from occupational therapist ■ Refer to Occupational Therapy sheet (**OT1**)
■ Accurate placement of objects/component parts in relation to size/length/depth/height when free drawing or copying	■ Explore properties of finished product prior to drawing Discuss properties of component parts in relation to the whole Divide paper into squares and provide positional references	
■ Neatness and presentation of drawings	■ Try using alternative medium, e.g. chalk, pastels Choose activity carefully to enhance student's ability to succeed Divide paper into squares and provide positional reference	
■ Construction tasks	■ Use alternative materials, e.g. sturdy rather than flimsy Reduce the need for precision by using larger equipment Provide part-prepared model Provide adult support when accuracy is paramount Work on a larger scale	
Visual spatial relationships	**It may be necessary to seek advice from your SENCO in order to implement some of these approaches**	**Refer to visual spatial relationship skill sheet (F7)**
■ Using linear and vertical scanning	■ Reinforce working left to right, top to bottom Use right-angled paper guide Use clear/perspex ruler as a line tracker Use squared/isometric paper to help with placing, e.g. as a guide	■ Refer to Foundation skill sheet (**F5**), Appendix (**A4**)

Table 3.9 Art

Possible Classroom Problem	Possible Practical Approach	Further Advice via SENCO
Visual spatial relationships (continued)		**Refer to visual spatial relationship skill sheet (F7)**
■ Drawing 2D representation of 3D objects	■ Work on squared or isometric paper Provide visual instructions on how to transfer 3D to 2D Teach 'rules' on how to draw common forms Allow time to plan and discuss spatial components of form/objects Use a multi-sensory approach, e.g. feeling, touching, verbalizing about artefact/item	
■ Understanding relationship between size, position, orientation of objects/forms	■ Allow time to plan and discuss spatial components of form/object Reinforce teaching of perspectives Use ruler, graph paper as visual cue of size, position, orientation	
■ Constructing models	■ Give concrete examples Reinforce spatial orientation of model, sculpture, collage Make prototype and discuss spatial aspects of form Reproduce instructions so each stage of process is visually represented	
■ Presentation and layout of work	■ Use appropriate computer software, e.g. Clip Art™, scanner Use of line/squared/graph paper Provide proforma with suggested layout	
Visual figure ground discrimination	**It may be necessary to seek advice from your SENCO in order to implement some of these approaches**	**Refer to visual figure ground skill sheet (F9)**
■ Preparation for lesson in general – finding appropriate equipment	■ Ensure work surfaces are clear Reinforce need to return equipment, e.g. pens, brushes, clay to allocated storage area after use Provide working surface which gives good contrast to assist with sorting/finding Limit the amount of information on a page/board and use different colours to highlight key information	

Occupational Therapy Approaches for Secondary Special Needs © Whurr Publishers Ltd 2002

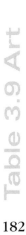

Possible Classroom Problem	Possible Practical Approach	Further Advice via SENCO
Visual figure ground discrimination (continued)		
■ Exploring specific detail within artistic forms, images and artefacts	■ Use a multi-sensory approach, e.g. feeling, touching, verbalizing Use of appropriate-sized window or magnifying glass to isolate a specific area	
■ Focusing on specific detail in order to copy an artistic form	■ Ensure artistic form is placed against a contrasting background Target overall shape/outline before working on specific detail	■ Refer to Foundation skill sheet **(F5)**
■ Finding appropriate equipment	■ Ensure items are stored correctly and clearly labelled Provide surface which gives a good contrast	
■ Cutting materials accurately, e.g. seeing line on material	■ Draw thicker/darker line or use a contrasting colour Provide adult support when accuracy or safety paramount Provide template in a contrasting colour to cut around Provide a safety ruler	
■ Seeing and recognizing artefacts on display in museums, galleries, etc.	■ Use buddy working/adult support Provide pictorial cue cards to match with artefact	
■ Selecting information using ICT, e.g. sites on internet screen	■ Heighten staff awareness to students difficulties Use buddy working/adult support Explain layout of information on screen Ensure student is familiar with software	
■ Organization and layout of overlapping drawings	■ Accentuate colour contrasts Use clear, uncluttered, part-prepared work sheets to limit drawing Allow student to trace drawings from text book	

Occupational Therapy Approaches for Secondary Special Needs © Whurr Publishers Ltd 2002

Possible Classroom Problem	Possible Practical Approach	Further Advice via SENCO
Visual form constancy	**It may be necessary to seek advice from your SENCO in order to implement some of these approaches**	**Refer to visual form constancy skill sheet (F8)**
■ Understanding and generalizing the common properties of a form/artefact, e.g. cup is a still cup regardless of size, shape, texture, colour	■ Use a multi-sensory approach, e.g. feeling, touching, verbalizing to investigate properties of the item Use cue cards listing essential properties Discuss common properties of form/artefact Reinforce concepts by analysing other students work	
■ Investigating and classifying art/craft/design in a variety of genres, styles and traditions	■ Heighten teachers' awareness of student's difficulties Provide checklist listing common properties	
■ Recognizing and using 2D representation of 3D object, e.g. a drawing of a cup represents the actual cup	■ Relate properties of drawing to concrete object	
Visual closure	**It may be necessary to seek advice from your SENCO in order to implement some of these approaches**	**Refer to visual closure skill sheet (F10)**
■ Being able to visualize completed art form	■ Discuss expected outcome before starting work Talk through each stage of process in relation to finished project Cue cards to ensure all aspects of completed art form are considered Use cue cards to identify each stage of the process, itemize component parts	
■ Developing and making an art form	■ Talk through ideas step by step Provide a step-by-step recipe Use mind-mapping techniques	
■ Identifying and locating objects on a crowded table/work bench when only part is visible	■ Maintain a clear, organized work surface	■ Refer to Further reading

Possible Classroom Problem	Possible Practical Approach	Further Advice via SENCO
Visual memory/visual sequential memory	**It may be necessary to seek advice from your SENCO in order to implement some of these approaches**	**Refer to visual memory/sequential memory skill sheet (F11)**
■ Copying from the board/book	■ Reduce copying from board, e.g. use part-prepared work sheets or give own copy of board information Check student's position in class – relative to board, position near and facing board Be aware of objects, in line of vision, which could interfere with student's view Try e.g. using stickers or different coloured pens as visual markers or to differentiate sections of text to be copied. Give adequate time for student to record work Place material to be copied in front of student – experiment with angle of surface to find optimum position	■ Refer to Foundation skill sheet (F5), Appendix (A4)
■ Remembering details of practical demonstration	■ Take notes during demonstration, e.g. pictorial, shorthand, prompt words and number points Break down each task and record each stage of process, e.g. using digital camera, numbered pictorial cue cards Use headings as a memory cues, e.g. items to collect Highlight each stage on instruction sheet or notes Use 'writing frames'	■ Refer to Further reading
■ Recording stages of art process	■ Encourage student to take notes on each stage as they are working Take photographs of each stage Use mind-mapping techniques	■ Refer to Further reading
Auditory processing and memory	**It may be necessary to seek advice from your SENCO in order to implement some of these approaches**	**Refer to auditory processing and memory skill sheet (F12)**
■ Following and remembering verbal instructions	■ Use dictaphone Use other senses to support auditory cues Give clear, concise instructions in small steps Repeat instructions, allowing student to verbalize back to check that they have heard and understood	■ Seek advice from speech and language therapist

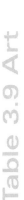

Table 3.9 Art

Possible Classroom Problem	Possible Practical Approach	Further Advice via SENCO
Auditory processing and memory (continued)		
■ Following and remembering verbal instructions (continued)	■ Reinforce with written notes and visual cues If possible withdraw student to quiet area and give assistance Use 'work schedules'	■ Refer to Appendix (**A5**)
■ Group discussion, e.g. ability to sift, summarise, use salient points, cite evidence	■ Frequent resumé of essential points by group leader Encourage student to record main points and write down any questions during discussion Ask student leading questions as a prompt Allow extra time for student to answer Use mind-mapping techniques	■ Seek advice from educational psychologist, speech and language specialist ■ Refer to Further reading
Social interaction	**It may be necessary to seek advice from your SENCO in order to implement some of these approaches**	**Refer to social interaction skill sheet (F13)**
■ Low self-esteem leading to withdrawal	■ Build student's confidence by breaking down task and concentrating on one aspect of the task Appropriate/fair use of praise	
■ Reluctance to handle certain materials due to tactile sensitivity leading to an inappropriate response	■ Consider use of alternative materials Wear surgical gloves	
■ Impulsiveness	■ Heighten teacher's and peers' awareness of student's difficulty Select group members carefully Ensure student has uncluttered work area Provide adult support Undertake risk assessment	■ Seek advice from school health and safety representative
■ Awareness of personal space (own and others)	■ Social skills training programme Heighten teachers' and peers' awareness of student's difficulties	■ Seek advice from educational psychologist, child and family adolescent mental health team
■ Working as part of a group	■ Select group members carefully Allocate achievable task to student Consider adult facilitation	

Occupational Therapy Approaches for Secondary Special Needs © Whurr Publishers Ltd 2002

CA9 Art

CA10

Table 3.10 Music

Possible Classroom Problem	Possible Practical Approach	Further Advice via SENCO
Gross motor co-ordination	**It may be necessary to liaise with your SENCO in order to implement some of these approaches**	**Refer to gross motor skill sheet (F1)**
Reduced stamina to maintain a functional playing position	■ Carefully consider choice of instrument Ensure optimum supported playing position is used Check position of music stand in relation to head position	
Ability to maintain functional writing posture	■ Check sitting posture – chair/table size and height Consider working on an angled surface, e.g. clipboard, lever-arch file	■ Refer to Occupational Therapy sheet (**OT1**) and Equipment resources (**ER**)
Grading for precision of movement to produce accurate sound	■ Practise to reinforce with auditory feedback, e.g. awareness of correct pitch/sound/volume	
Unable to maintain appropriate breath control	■ Teach breathing exercises Reinforce with auditory feedback	
Sustaining accurate timing when conducting	■ Improve shoulder strength through liaison with PE department Ensure optimum supported conducting position is used Consider trying different weighted batons	■ Refer to Occupational Therapy sheet (**OT6**)
Achieving accurate conducting patterns	■ Accentuate conducting pattern and reinforce with visual clues	
Mobility around the classroom	■ Keep pathways clear Remind students to store music cases appropriately	
Carrying musical instrument	■ Select an appropriate instrument Provide storage for instrument Use buddy working/adult support	
Ability to set up equipment	■ Use buddy working/adult support Consider choice of equipment	

CA10

Table 3.10 Music

Possible Classroom Problem	Possible Practical Approach	Further Advice via SENCO
Gross motor co-ordination (continued)		
■ Anchoring and stabilizing equipment	■ Select an appropriate instrument Explore accessories available to support instrument	■ Seek advice from head of music
Fine motor dexterity	**It may be necessary to liaise with your SENCO in order to implement some of these approaches**	**Refer to fine motor dexterity skill sheet (F2)**
■ Accuracy for e.g. musical notation	■ Use manuscript paper Try enlarging manuscript paper Trial of different writing tools Use buddy working/adult support as a scribe	■ Refer to Occupational Therapy sheet (**OT1**) and Equipment resources (**ER**)
■ Assembling instrument	■ Use buddy working/adult support Keep instrument assembled for as long as possible	
■ Positioning fingers on instrument	■ Practise hand strengthening, finger isolation, tactile awareness exercises Carefully consider choice of instrument	■ Refer to Occupational Therapy sheet (**OT5**)
■ Cleaning and disassembling instruction	■ Use buddy working/adult support	
Organizational skills	**It may be necessary to liaise with your SENCO in order to implement some of these approaches**	**Refer to organizational skill sheet (F3)**
■ Correct positioning of fingers/body in order to produce precise note	■ Colour code instrument One-to-one explanation	■ Seek advice from the head of music
■ Assembling instrument, music stand	■ Diagrammatic guide, cue card Use colour-coding system Use buddy working/adult support Consider choice of instrument	

Possible Classroom Problem	Possible Practical Approach	Further Advice via SENCO
Organizational skills (continued)		
■ Ability to find place on music sheet	■ Use buddy working/adult support	
■ Sequencing, timing and rhythm	■ Provide additional cueing from leader/conductor Use metronome Accentuate conducting pattern and reinforce with visual cues	
■ Reading and interpreting music	■ Cue card for musical terms Extra practice and over-learning	
■ Composing and combining musical resources	■ Select appropriate group members who are musically competent	
■ Creating ideas, conceptualization and initiating original thought	■ Use mind-mapping techniques Buddy working with a competent student	■ Refer to Further reading
■ Using ICT equipment	■ One-to-one explanation Use of cue cards/diagrammatic step-by-step guide on how to set up and use equipment Ensure student is familiar with software	
■ Organizing work area	■ Consider providing student with extra space Define allocated work area Consider use of 'work schedules' Encourage student to store equipment appropriately	■ Refer to Appendix (**A5**)

Table 3.10 Music

Possible Classroom Problem	Possible Practical Approach	Further Advice via SENCO
Visual motor integration	**It may be necessary to liaise with your SENCO in order to implement some of these approaches**	**Refer to visual motor integration skill skeet (F6)**
■ Accurate manipulative skills when playing instruments leading to poor note production	■ Choose instrument carefully to enhance success Colour code instrument for accurate placement of fingers Ensure optimum supportive e.g. playing position is used	
■ Following conductor whilst playing instrument	■ Heighten staff awareness of student's difficulty Consider pairing with a more able student	
■ Interpreting musical notation	■ Highlight musical notation on music sheet	
Visual spatial relationships	**It may be necessary to liaise with your SENCO in order to implement some of these approaches**	**Refer to visual spatial relationship skill skeet (F7)**
■ Writing musical notations on the correct line	■ Use appropriate ICT to write music Enlarge manuscript paper Increase contrast on paper Use buddy working/adult support	■ Seek advice from ICT advisor, refer to Appendix (A3) ■ Seek advice from head of music
■ Accurate spacing and sizing of notations	■ Use appropriate ICT to write music Use buddy working/adult support	
■ Linear scanning to read and interpret music	■ Compensate through using another sense, e.g. aural learning	■ Refer to Foundation skill sheet (F5), Appendix (A4)
■ Quick localization – when finding place in music	■ Over-learning to familarize self with piece Conductor's awareness of student's difficulty	

Possible Classroom Problem	Possible Practical Approach	Further Advice via SENCO
Visual figure ground discrimination	**It may be necessary to liaise with your SENCO in order to implement some of these approaches**	**Refer to visual figure ground skill sheet (F9)**
■ Reading music	■ Enlarge manuscript Increase contrast between paper and notation Try colour overlays	■ Refer to Foundation skill sheet (F5)
■ Positioning fingers whilst learning instruments	■ Colour code position of notes on instrument Practise in front of a mirror 'Parallel' playing beside teacher or an able student	
■ Assembling musical instrument	■ Highlight parts of instrument which fit together, e.g with tape, stickers Adult support/buddy working	
■ Assembling and using ICT equipment	■ Code/colour code plugs, leads, etc. Adult support/buddy working Provide step-by-step diagrammatic instruction, colour coded to correspond with colours used on plugs, leads	
Visual form constancy	**It may be necessary to liaise with your SENCO in order to implement some of these approaches**	**Refer to visual form constancy skill sheet (F8)**
■ Recognizing that note values change according to how they are written	■ Heighten staff awareness	
Visual closure	**It may be necessary to liaise with your SENCO in order to implement some of these approaches**	**Refer to visual closure skill sheet (F10)**
■ Fluency for reading music	■ Highlight phrases, patterns, chords Check frequently that musical notation is understood Use auditory methods to reinforce visual patterns/timing	

CA10 Music (continued)

Table 3.10 Music

Possible Classroom Problem	Possible Practical Approach	Further Advice via SENCO
Visual memory/sequential memory	**It may be necessary to liaise with your SENCO in order to implement some of these approaches**	**Refer to visual memory/sequential memory skills sheet (F11)**
Remembering musical sequences or words in songs	■ Have music/words available whenever possible Use auditory methods to reinforce visual patterns/timing	
Inability to look at conductor and music/words simultaneously	■ Heighten conductor's awareness of student's difficulty Consider position of student within group	■ Refer to Appendix (**A1**)
Copying music/words from board/book	■ Reduce copying from board/book, e.g. use pre-prepared worksheets, give student a copy of the information Check student's position relative to board, ensure nothing between student and board to interfere with vision Give adequate time for student to record work Place information in a vertical plane by using music stand	■ Refer to Foundation skill sheet (**F5**)
Auditory processing and memory	**It may be necessary to liaise with your SENCO in order to implement some of these approaches**	**Refer to auditory processing and memory skill skeet (F12)**
Listen and repeating sequence of sounds	■ Break down into small phrases and practise	■ Seek advice from head of music and speech and language therapist
Listening, judging and reproducing sound intervals	■ Work on internal visualization using cue cards, actual instruments	
Discriminating variation of sound, tone, rhythm and speed	■ Work one to one with an adult to break down into component notes and practice	
Ability to listen and reproduce musical phrases	■ Use a multi-sensory approach, e.g. look, clap, listen	
Remembering words of songs	■ Have words available	

Occupational Therapy Approaches for Secondary Special Needs © Whurr Publishers Ltd 2002

Possible Classroom Problem	Possible Practical Approach	Further Advice via SENCO
	It may be necessary to liaise with your SENCO in order to implement some of these approaches	**Refer to social interaction skill sheet (F13)**
Social interaction		
■ Hypersensitivity to sound producing an extreme, unacceptable response, e.g. hands over ears, leaving the room	■ Awareness of student's physical discomfort Prepare student for increased sound level Use headphones to dampen noise	■ Seek advice from speech and language therapist, occupational therapist
■ Low self-esteem leading to withdrawal	■ Build student's confidence by breaking down tasks and setting achievable goals	
■ Inability to pick up appropriate cues within musical group work	■ Social skills training Exaggerate cues	■ Seek advice from child and adolescent mental health services, educational pyschologist
■ Impulsiveness	■ Give student object to 'fiddle' with when not performing a specific task Heighten teachers' and peers' awareness of student's difficulty Select group members carefully Consider choice of instrument carefully	

CA11

Table 3.11 Physical education

CAUTION
When a student has been diagnosed with a specific medical condition please ensure that you have read the relevant table in the conditions chapter prior to planning an activity. If a physiotherapist is involved it is essential to liaise with the therapist since damage could occur through inappropriate activities.

Possible Classroom Problem	Possible Practical Approach	Further Advice via SENCO
Gross motor co-ordination	**It may be necessary to seek advice from your SENCO in order to implement some of these approaches**	**Refer to gross motor co-ordination skill sheet (F1)**

■ Muscle tone
  (a) low/floppy (hypotonic):
    props/flops (against students/floor/furniture)
    poor stamina and difficulty sustaining movements
    unable to accelerate/decelerate quickly or to make sharp
      directional changes
    heavy, 'earthbound' movements
    poor grading of movements
    instability in balance/counterbalance activities
    constant movement to give themselves stability
    difficulty maintaining control of movement
    difficulty with rhythmic/synchronization work
    poor competence in ball/target skills
    falls frequently
    reluctance to participate due to anticipated difficulties
	■ Choose activities carefully to enhance student's
	    ability to succeed
	  Pre-select groups to ensure compatibility of
	    partner/opponent
	  Use smaller/lighter weight equipment
	  Involve in team support activities, e.g.
	    equipment monitors, linesmen, referee
	  Introduce carefully graded programme of motor
	    activities to improve muscle strength
		■ Seek advice from PE advisor,
		  physiotherapist, occupational
		  therapist, advisory teacher,
		  school health and safety repre-
		  sentative
		
		■ Refer to Occupational Therapy
		  sheet (**OT6**); James Russell's
		  Graded Motor Activities and
		  Elphinston Pook, *The Core
		  Workout*

Warning: It is essential to refer to section on cerebral palsy (pp. 55–65) and liaise with the physiotherapist since damage can occur through inappropriate activities		

(b) high/spasticity (hypertonic):
    instability in balance/counterbalance activities
    poor competence in ball/target skills
    poor stamina and difficulty sustaining movements
    poor grading/movements
    lack of fluency of movements
    difficulty with sharp directional changes
	■ Choose activity carefully to reduce potential
	    for increasing tone
	  Investigate alternative options, e.g. team
	    support activities, practising of other
	    skills (i.e. keyboard skills), community
	    service
	  Adapt the activity to improve student's
	    ability to participate
	  Pre-select groups to ensure compatibility
	    with partner/opponent
		■ Seek advice from physiotherapist,
		  PE advisor, advisory teacher,
		  sports disability advisor

CA11 Physical education (continued)

Possible Classroom Problem	Possible Practical Approach	Further Advice via SENCO
Postural instability props/flops (against wall/children/furniture) assumes a fixed flexion position lacks fluency of movement difficulty accelerating/decelerating ungainly/awkward/exaggerated movements reduced ability with hopping, balance, changing direction difficulty with rhythmic/synchronized movements	■ Choose activity carefully to enhance student's ability to succeed, e.g. swimming Introduce carefully graded strengthening programme to improve stability Grade rhythm from relatively slow and allow prolonged period at same rhythm before changing Start with small angle of directional change and increase angle as ability improves Heighten teachers' awareness of safety implications and consider need for a risk assessment	■ Refer to Occupational Therapy sheet (**OT6**); James Russell's *Graded Motor Activities* and Elphinston Pook, *The Core Workout*. Seek advice from PE advisor, physiotherapist, occupational therapist, advisory teacher, school health and safety representative
Balance difficulty executing precise controlled movements, e.g. in gym/dance difficulty in counterbalance activities appears awkward/uncoordinated uses speed in an attempt to overcome poor balance dislike/anxiety over apparatus work falls frequently	■ Carefully graded programme to improve control Use static activities to encourage student to slow down Choose activity carefully to enhance student's ability to succeed Heighten teachers' awareness of safety implications and consider need for a risk assessment	
Bilateral skills poor accuracy in bat-and-ball games difficulty executing movements requiring co-ordination of the body, e.g. swimming with recognized strokes, athletics, gymnastics, dance	■ Break down movement into component parts and teach parts through regular practice with a competent partner Movement shadowing of a competent partner	
Proprioception lack e.g. of fluency and poor control of movements (grading) whole body co-ordination affected reduced spatial awareness bumping into, hitting equipment/peers without intent constant movement in an attempt to raise own body awareness awareness of body position and movement when unable to visually monitor body movements, e.g. swimming poor ball skills and bat-ball co-ordination	■ Increase body awareness through graded/resisted activities, e.g. trampoline, weight training, Increase peers' awareness of student's difficulty Reduce size of playing/target areas Use lightweight 'slow' balls Practise catching/throwing with a competent partner Introduce carefully graded strengthening programme	

Table 3.11 Physical education

Possible Classroom Problem	Possible Practical Approach	Further Advice via SENCO
Fine motor dexterity	**It may be necessary to seek advice from your SENCO in order to implement some of these approaches**	**Refer to fine motor dexterity skill sheet (F2)**
■ Holding and maintaining correct grasp on equipment dance – ribbons athletics – javelin/shot gymnastics – rings/rope general games – bats/hockey stick/ball	■ Consider trying equipment of different weights Experiment with different sizes/texture handles Mark position for correct grasp, e.g. tape/sweatband around handle Use general hand strengthening activities Consider alternative activities not requiring sustained grasps	■ Seek advice from PE advisor, advisory teachers, occupational therapist ■ Refer to Occupational Therapy sheet (**OT5**)
■ Changing for PE managing/fastenings/laces (unable to do or not tight enough) slower than peers untidy appearance, e.g. buttons/laces undone extra difficulty after showering if dressing whilst damp	■ Discuss with student and parents the possibility of trying alternative clothing with few buttons/adapting clothing with velcro fastenings/using elastic/curly laces Provide adult support Allow student extra time Allocate sufficient space within changing area	
■ Using specific equipment, e.g. compass, stopwatch, measuring tape	■ Explore alternative equipment	
■ Difficulty with ball skills, e.g. catching	■ Allocate to a competent group/partner who can give good feed back and catch difficult throws Give balance of a contrasting activity which the student is more competent at, e.g. running, creative work	
■ Bilateral activities where each hand is performing a different movement e.g. placing ball to serve in tennis	■ Focus on practising components of movement before requiring the whole movement, e.g. practise ball release with a preparatory racket swing	■ Seek advice from PE advisor, advisory teachers, occupational therapist
Organizational skills	**It may be necessary to seek advice from your SENCO in order to implement some of these approaches**	**Refer to organizational skill sheet (F3)**
■ Remembering and executing sequences of movement, e.g. athletics, gym, dance, swimming	■ Extra practice and repetition to overlearn/reinforce movement patterns and 'motor memory' for activity Use prompts, either visual or auditory	

Possible Classroom Problem	Possible Practical Approach	Further Advice via SENCO
Organizational skills (continued)		
■ Creating and performing own movement sequences	■ Practise individual sequences before linking together Choose group members carefully	
■ Remembering appropriate PE kit	■ Use a checklist Liaise with parents – try a pictorial timetable	■ Refer to Occupational Therapy sheet (**OT7**)
■ Changing/dressing for PE/games	■ Provide adult support Provide physical/verbal prompt for orientation of clothes Discuss need to practise dressing sequences at home with parents and student	
■ Understanding rules/tactics/strategies of team games	■ Consider multi-sensory approach to teach rules, e.g. visual, auditory, use of video Learn through continued practice and explanation Limit possible positions student learns so they develop awareness of that specific role on team	
■ Following verbal instructions	■ Use prompt/cue cards	■ Seek advice from speech and language therapist
■ Organization of self around pitch/circuit/track	■ Carefully consider type of sport chosen as it may be easier to learn a set layout, e.g. athletics, swimming, cricket Limit positions student learns so they develop awareness of that specific role on team Use lines/static markers as reference points Consider use of colour to assist organisation, e.g. colour band around goal post	

■ Outdoor adventure activities
    map reading
    orienteering
    problem-solving
	■ Extra practice and repetition
	Consider use of checklists for equipment
	Consider use of colour coding cues on map, e.g. top
	Break down instructions given
	Have 'map key' with symbols readily available
	Explain basic map features, e.g. contours
	Use buddy working/adult support	

■ Difficulty timing response in relation to speed, direction and distance	■ Break down task and practice component skills Consider alternative activity	

Occupational Therapy Approaches for Secondary Special Needs © Whurr Publishers Ltd 2002   **CA11 Physical education** (continued)

CA11

Table 3.11 Physical education

Possible Classroom Problem	Possible Practical Approach	Further Advice via SENCO
Visual motor integration	**It may be necessary to seek advice from your SENCO in order to implement some of these approaches**	**Refer to visual motor integration skill sheet (F6)**
■ Following flight of ball for catching	■ Reinforce eye to ball co-ordination by practising solo skills, e.g. bouncing ball on floor and catching on rebound, throwing ball against wall and catching after a bounce Start with large light balls or bean bags, build up towards smaller, heavier balls Ensure student works with a competent partner Encourage participation in sports which do not require catching	■ Refer to Foundation skill sheet (**F5**)
■ Hitting target	■ Extra practice/over-learning of skill/activity Where possible allow student to perform practice shots first Start with large, close target and then gradually reduce distance/size Observe successful target range and utilize, then use this successful target range with different size/weights of balls	■ Seek advice from PE advisor, advisory teacher, physiotherapist, occupational therapist
Visual spatial relationships	**It may be necessary to seek advice from your SENCO in order to implement some of these approaches**	**Refer to visual spatial relationship foundation skill sheet (F7)**
■ Finding, maintaining and relocating correct position on pitch, court, field	■ Limit number of playing positions student is taught Reinforce boundary areas on pitch, court, etc. Use lines/static markers as a reference point Carefully consider type of sport chosen as it may be easier to learn a sport with a set pitch/court layout, e.g. athletics, swimming, cricket	■ Refer to Foundation skill sheet (**F5**)
■ Negotiating self within space and in relation to other students	■ Carefully consider type of sporting activity Avoid activities which have fast and unpredictable changes in direction.	

CA11 Physical education (continued)

Possible Classroom Problem	Possible Practical Approach	Further Advice via SENCO
Visual spatial relationships (continued)		
■ Negotiating self within space and in relation to other students (continued)	■ Consider activities where there are consistent points of reference	
■ Exaggerated 'clumsiness' when wearing protective clothing/footwear due to inability to adjust body awareness	■ Heighten teacher/peer awareness Decide whether it is imperative for student to wear protective clothing/footwear	■ Refer to school health and safety policy/representative
■ Judging distances	■ Provide concrete frame of reference, e.g. marker Extra practice and over-learning of the specific skill/activity	
■ Correct perception of height and depth	■ Consider if appropriate for student to participate Extra practice and over-learning of the skill/activity Provide adult support	■ Refer to school health and safety policy
■ Performing quick directional changes	■ Choose games with reduced need to make changes Choose activities where directional changes can be pre-planned or activities which have a slower pace and practice	
Visual form constancy	**It may be necessary to seek advice from your SENCO in order to implement some of these approaches**	**Refer to visual form constancy skill sheet (F8)**
■ Recognizing different apparatus, e.g. in gymnastics, when seen from different angles	■ Discuss and reinforce recognition of equipment from different angles	
■ Recognizing that an individual's playing position, e.g. defender remains constant, although their action position on field/pitch may be changed	■ Consider alternative PE options which limit the number of seemingly random movements, e.g. athletics, table tennis Use of numbered vest/shirts	
■ Selecting equipment from a store when it is seen from an unusual angle	■ Increase staff awareness of student's difficulty Use a buddy working system	

Occupational Therapy Approaches for Secondary Special Needs © Whurr Publishers Ltd 2002

CA11 Physical education (continued)

Table 3.11 Physical education

Possible Classroom Problem	Possible Practical Approach	Further Advice via SENCO
Visual figure ground discrimination	**It may be necessary to seek advice from your SENCO in order to implement some of these approaches**	**Refer to visual figure ground skill sheet (F9)**
■ Locating and adhering to relevant markings on multi-purpose courts	■ Reinforce colour of markings for game being played Where possible use court/pitch which is dedicated to only one sport Consider environment, sun, orientation of play	
■ Picking out ball, etc. from background ■ Reading and interpreting information on a map, e.g. orienteering	■ Ensure good colour contrast ■ Choose alternative activity Use buddy working/adult support Consider need for risk assessment	■ Refer to school health and safety policy
Visual closure	**It may be necessary to seek advice from your SENCO in order to implement some of these approaches**	**Refer to visual closure skill sheet (F10)**
■ Recognizing equipment in PE store when only part of a object is visible, e.g. hockey stick from part-visible handle	■ Increase staff awareness of student's difficulty Use labelling	
■ Keeping score/refereeing ■ Recognizing developments of movement patterns, e.g. scrum, dance	■ Provide adult/peer support ■ Regular practice	
Visual memory/sequential memory	**It may be necessary to seek advice from your SENCO in order to implement some of these approaches**	**Refer to visual memory/sequential memory skill sheet (F11)**
■ Remembering order of equipment in a circuit	■ Reinforce sequence Use a card numbering system Use a buddy working system – shadowing a competent student	
■ Remembering dance routines and sequences of movement, e.g. aerobics	■ Over-learning of routines/movement sequences Use other senses to assist, e.g. auditory cues	
■ Ability to assume standard postures from memory	■ Regular practice Shadowing of adult/competent student	
■ Copying or imitating others	■ Ensure student is directly in front of teacher Choose options which are either slower or require less imitation	

Occupational Therapy Approaches for Secondary Special Needs © Whurr Publishers Ltd 2002

CA11 Physical education (continued)

Possible Classroom Problem	Possible Practical Approach	Further Advice via SENCO
Auditory processing and memory	**It may be necessary to seek advice from your SENCO in order to implement some of these approaches**	**Refer to auditory processing and memory skill sheet (F12)**
■ Following/remembering instructions	■ Give clear concise instructions Ask student/class to repeat instructions Use cue cards	
■ Slow response to instructions in team situations	■ Heighten peers' awareness of student's difficulty Allow familiarization in one playing position	
■ Recalling sequence of events, e.g. gymnastics, dance routines	■ Repeat instructions and allow students to verbalize back to check she or he has heard and understood them Use written checklist Encourage student/class to verbalize as performing movements Use buddy working/adult support	■ Seek advice from speech and language therapist
Social interaction	**It may be necessary to seek advice from your SENCO in order to implement some of these approaches**	**Refer to social interaction skill sheet (F13)**
■ Awareness of team roles, team working	■ Consider multi-sensory approach to teach rules, e.g. visual, auditory, use of video	
■ Awareness of appropriate social behaviour in team sports	■ Choose alternative activity which is less socially demanding Behavioural management programme	
■ Failure to initiate contact with others	■ Carefully select team members who will initiate contact with student Social skills training programme	■ Seek advice from educational psychologist, child and adolescent mental health service, speech and language therapist, health and safety representative
■ Low self-esteem and awareness of failure	■ Build up confidence by breaking down tasks and setting achievable goals. Consider alternative options to PE Reward effort as well as achievement	
■ Impulsiveness	■ Heighten awareness for safety issues	

Chapter 4

Occupational Therapy Skills Sheets

Introduction

These Occupational Therapy skill sheets, give practical suggestions which can be incorporated into the student's individual education plan (IEP). It is recognized that teachers in school are not trained to devise occupational therapy programmes. However, in light of the fact that few secondary schools have access to occupational therapists, these sheets have been written to enable the ideas to be implemented by any staff without formal occupational therapy training.

OT1 Posture/handwriting/pencil and paper tasks

Functional sitting position

It is important that the student sits correctly so that he or she can concentrate on the classroom task without having to be constantly aware of his or her physical position. The student who is not positioned correctly will use increased effort to maintain good sitting balance to the detriment of precision for fine motor or cognitive tasks.

As a quick rule of thumb, seat heights should be at least one-third of the student's height. Seats should have a forward sloping angle and the table should be at least half the student's height.

Students may be helped to adopt a good sitting position by ensuring:

- **feet are supported** – flat on the floor or on a footrest;
- **knees are at 90°**;
- **chair seat depth** will fully support thighs;
- **lower trunk is touching the back of chair**;
- **student leans slightly forward** – optimum position 30° from upright;
- **forearms on the table**;
- **head is up** - approximate distance from table is elbow joint to the middle knuckle;
- **chair is pulled into the table/desk**;
- **table height** – approx 5 cm above the level of student's bent elbow when seated as above;
- an **angled writing surface** is available if required;
- **elbows are resting on the table** in a comfortable position (at least 30° from body).

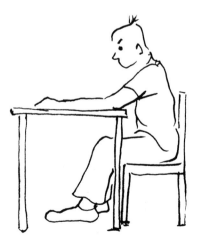

Figure 4.1 Correct sitting position

Functional working position in standing

Students who have difficulty maintaining an upright standing posture will find fine motor tasks hard since they are needing to focus and concentrate on maintaining working posture.

Students who cannot maintain an upright position may be helped by:

- **allowing student to lean (prop)** against an appropriate fixed work surface;
- **enlarging student's workspace** to allow for propping and excess movements;
- **providing a high stool** with footrest or perching stool;
- **checking height of the table/bench**, i.e. 5 cm above elbow;
- **providing a raised platform** if bench is too high;
- **sitting for task** or providing a raised table if table/bench is too low;
- **adapting task** to enable student to sit throughout;
- **using a folding/camping stool** or shooting stick on field trips;
- **alternating standing with sitting;**
- **ensuring music stand is at correct height** relative to student thus maintaining optimum visual field and maintaining head/body alignment.

Table surface

It is essential that the writing surface is relatively clear so that the student can concentrate on the task without distractions. The table surface may need to be angled to provide:

- a more efficient position;
- stability of shoulders to increase handwriting flow;
- easier visual focus.

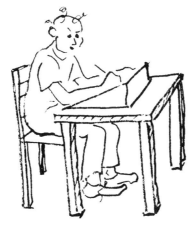

Figure 4.2 Working at angled surface

Students may be helped to work in a more efficient position by:

- **experimenting with the gradient of working slope** required to achieve student's optimum working position. The recommended angle is 20°, however some students prefer more or less of an incline.

- **using commercially available angled surfaces** (see Equipment resources) or home-made model designed to the student's requirements;

- **improvizing angled surface** with a lever-arch file or clipboard resting against pencil case/book;

- **ensuring use of drawing board/easel** in appropriate lessons;

- **sitting appropriately;**

- **working on a non-slip surface.**

Texture of paper

It is important to use good quality paper which will not smudge or crease under the student's hand. The paper texture will affect the movement of the writing tool.

- **Shiny and glossy paper** will increase the fluency of the tool so is useful for students who have difficulty with smooth movements.

- **Matt and textured paper** provides more friction giving the student greater control of the writing tool.

Paper position

The position of the paper in relation to the student may affect the flow and speed of handwriting. Some students can produce good handwriting with paper in a variety of positions, but ideally:

- **right-handed students – angle paper to left**
- **left-handed students – angle paper to right**

An optimum position for paper is an angle between 35 and 45°. An easy method for achieving this is to get the student to:

- sit straight at table (check posture);

- clasp hands together in line with both head and midline of body, place forearms on table to make a triangle;

- lay paper parallel to writing hand inside the formed triangle.

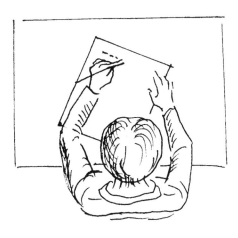

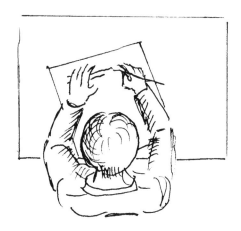

Figure 4.3 Left and right hand paper position

Pen/tool grasp

The student's tool grasp may affect the control efficiency, flow and speed of written output. An incorrect grasp may hinder the amount of recording a student is able to achieve before experiencing discomfort in the writing hand or forearm.

An efficient grasp, commonly referred to as a tripod grasp, consists of:

- holding shaft of pen between pads of index finger and thumb;
- supporting underside of tool shaft on side of middle finger, with ring and little finger slightly curled into palm to provide stability;
- resting outer surface of hand (little finger side) on writing surface.

A combination of finger and wrist movements allow the writer to control the tool and regulate the amount of pressure exerted. (See Figure 4.4 for the tripod grasp and Figures 4.5 and 4.6 for other efficient alternative grasps.)

An inefficient grasp does not allow the tool to be held securely to enable a fluid and smooth writing action. Some inefficient grasps are illustrated in Figures 4.7, 4.8, 4.9 and 4.10.

Efficient grasps

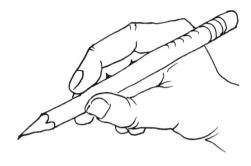

Figure 4.4 Tripod grasp

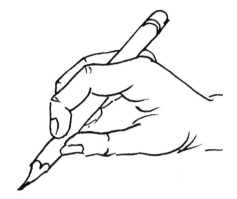

Figure 4.5 Adapted tripod grasp

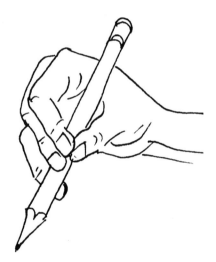

Figure 4.6 Quadrupod grasp

Inefficient grasps

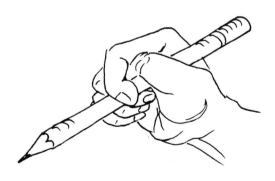

Figure 4.7 Thumb tuck grasp

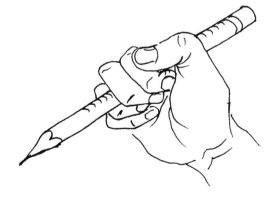

Figure 4.8 Interdigital brace grasp

Inefficient grasps (continued)

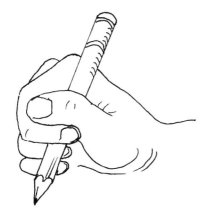

Figure 4.9 Thumb wrap grasp

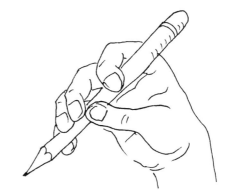

Figure 4.10 Index grasp

Pressure

A student's pen pressure affects his or her control, efficiency, flow and output. Heavy pressure results in:

- excessive strain on thumb, finger joints and forearm leading to pain;
- increased force on the end joint of index/middle finger causing an excessive dipped appearance (see Figure 4.11).

Heavy pressure causes:

- loss of fluency;
- increased tension in forearm and wrist;
- difficulty writing for a sustained period of time;
- paper becoming imprinted;
- holes being made in paper.

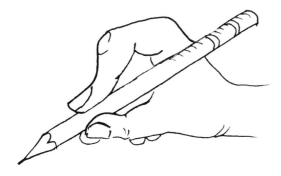

Figure 4.11 Tripod grasp with hyper-extension of index finger

OT1

Students who display heavy pressure may be helped by:

- **using an angled surface;**
- **using pencil/pen with larger barrel** to reduce strain on finger joints;
- **using commercially available pens with a cushioned grip** incorporated into the barrel;
- **investigating nib type and flow of pen on paper,** e.g. fountain pen, roller ball, fibre tip;
- **writing in an exercise book** rather than on a single sheet of paper on desk;
- **placing card under paper** to prevent imprint of text onto next page;
- **placing carpet tile under paper** so that the student can learn to adapt the amount of pressure exerted;
- **using hand relaxation techniques** (see occupational therapy sheet **OT4**).

Light pressure causes:

- poor pencil control;
- inability to make consistent marks on paper;
- illegible, spidery script.

Students who press lightly may be helped by:

- **using an angled surface** to improve functional posture;
- **investigating nib type and flow of pen on paper,** e.g. fibre tip, roller ball, fine flow soft pencils;
- **using hand strengthening activities** (see Occupational Therapy sheet **OT5**).

Changing a tool grasp at secondary level is extremely difficult and is dependent on the motivation of the student to attempt the task. When undertaken, it is essential that both teachers and support staff are aware that the student is attempting to improve his or her tool grasp and to provide positive help and feedback as required.

Students who are trying to change their tool grasp may be helped by:

- **regular opportunities to practise hand and upper body strengthening activities** (see occupational therapy sheets **OT5** and **OT6**);

- **trial of alternative pens** to determine the most comfortable and efficient with particular reference to:

  - **shaft/barrel size** – larger barrels open the student's web space and reduces tension;
  - **integral/cushion grip** – to help with placement of finger and thumb on shaft which may reduce tension of the pencil grasp;
  - **weight** – a heavy weight pen can help student dampen a tremor, a light weight pen can be helpful for student with muscle weakness;
  - **flow** – investigate properties of different pens, e.g. roller pens, fountain pen, felt tip, ballpoints, calligraphy pen.

Left-handed students may find a broader, more flexible nib will prevent them making holes in the paper or slowing unnecessarily.

References

Brown B, Henderson S (1989) A sloping desk? Should the wheel turn full circle? Handwriting Review No 3.

Henderson S, Markee A, Scheib B, Taylor J (1999) Tools of the Trade. Hemingford Abbot: Handwriting Interest Group.

Penso D (1990) Keyboard Graphics and Handwriting Skills. London: Chapman and Hall.

Shirley, M (1996) Why look at school furniture? Handwriting Review 10: 55-65.

Taylor J (2001) Handwriting. A Teacher's Guide. London: Fulton.

Other useful resources

Chu S (2000) The effects of visual perception: Dysfunctions on the development and performance of handwriting skills. Handwriting Today 2: 42-55.

Fagg R. Helping Left-handed Children Enjoy Handwriting. Available from Anything Left Handed Ltd (see Suppliers' Addresses).

Levine K (1991) Fine Motor Dysfunction – Therapeutic Strategies in the Classroom: Therapy Skill Builders. Tuscon, AZ: Therapy Skill Builders.

Pickard P (1987) Handwriting – A Second Chance (41 photocopy master worksheets for secondary pupils with handwriting difficulties). Wisbech: LDA Living and Learning.

Teodorescu I, Addy L (1997) Write from the Start. Wisbech: LDA Living and Learning.

OT2 Advice for left-handed students

Writing tool and grasp

In order to see the text as they write and prevent smudging, left-handed students should hold the pen/pencil at least 2cm from the point (see Figure 4.12). This can be indicated by a small elastic band around the desired area or by using a pen with an integral grip. A left-hander student often pushes the pen/pencil across the paper. Ballpoint, Berol or fibre tip pens produce less friction, whilst specially made left-hander nibs are available from commercial stationers.

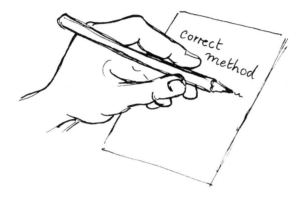

Figure 4.12 Correct grasp for left-handed student

Students who have already developed a hooked grip (Figure 4.13) are likely to experience:

- **reduced fluency** of arm and finger movements resulting in having to move the whole arm across the page;
- **jerky effortful movements** causing reduced speed of written output;

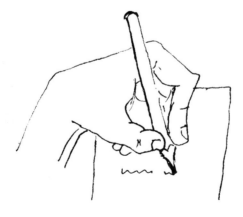

Figure 4.13 Hooked grasp

- **pain and fatigue in wrist and fingers** for extended periods of writing;
- **smudging of work** done due to covering up the previous lines of text;
- **difficulty achieving neat writing** and satisfactory presentation of work.

Students may be helped by:

- **using a sloping desk top**, resting work on a lever-arch file or a clipboard;
- **implementing relaxation techniques** (see Occupational Therapy sheet **OT4**);
- **experimenting with alternative tools**, pens or softer pencils;
- **ensuring paper is angled** correctly for a left-handed student.

Paper postition

The position of the paper in relation to the student will affect the flow and speed of handwriting. There are two coping strategies frequently seen within the classroom:

1 The student turns the paper completely sideways or writes down towards the body, which can cause smudging and puts strain on the shoulder joint (Figure 4.14).

2 The student places paper vertically in front of the body, which cramps the left hand into the side (Figure 4.15).

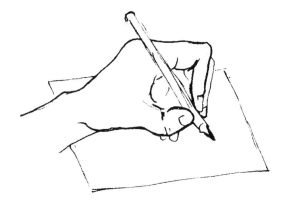

Figure 4.14

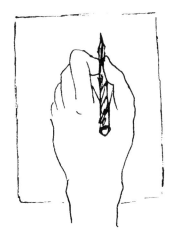

Figure 4.15

An optimum position for paper is at an angle of 35–45°. An easy method for achieving this is to get the student to angle the paper towards the right by:

- sitting straight at the table with correct posture (see Occupational Therapy sheet **OT1**);
- clasping hands together in line with both head and midline of body, placing forearms on the table to make a triangle;
- moving the whole triangle to left of midline so hands are in front of the left shoulder
- laying paper parallel to left arm inside formed triangle.

The paper should be far enough to the left to enable the student to rest his or her elbow on the working surface and move the forearm in an arc without crossing the body. Position the left hand below the writing line to enable the student to see what is being written. The paper position may need adjusting.

Sitting position

Students may be helped to adopt a good sitting position by ensuring:

- **feet are supported** – flat on the floor or on a footrest;
- **knees are at 90°**;
- **chair seat depth** will fully support thighs;
- **lower trunk is touching the back of the chair**;
- **student leans slightly forward** – optimum position 30° from upright;
- **forearms on the table**;
- **head is up** – approximate distance from table is elbow joint to the middle knuckle;
- **chair is pulled into the table/desk**;
- **table height** – approx 5 cm above the level of student's bent elbow when seated as above;
- that an **angled writing surface** is available;
- **elbows are resting on the table** in a comfortable position (at least 30° from body).

To avoid their arms colliding, ensure that a left-handed student is not sitting too close to a right-handed student. Check that light is coming over the right shoulder to avoid casting shadows on the work.

Occupational Therapy Approaches for Secondary Special Needs © Whurr Publishers Ltd 2002

OT2

Useful resources

215

The following resources are available from Anything Left Handed, (see Supplier's addresses page 246)

- Writing Left Handed
- Helping Left Handed Children to Enjoy Handwriting
- Left Handed Children – A Guide for Teachers and Parents
- The Left Hander's Handbook

OT3 Rules for writing tasks

Preparation for writing tasks

Before starting any written work think:

Posture

Pencil

Paper

Pressure

Presser

Posture:
- bottom at the back of the chair
- knees at right angles
- feet flat on the floor
- head and trunk leaning slightly forward
- hands and forearms on the table/chair well pushed in
- head at the distance from the desk of the knuckles to elbows

Pencil:
- functional grasp

Paper:
- angled to the left if tool in right hand
- angled to the right if tool in left hand

Pressure:
- even pressure – not too light nor too heavy

Presser:
- use presser (piece of stiff card) to write on

Occupational Therapy Approaches for Secondary Special Needs © Whurr Publishers Ltd 2002

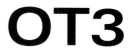

Success of writing task

Evaluate letters for

Shape

Slope

Size

Spacing

Sitting on line

Shape:

- are the letter shapes correct?

Slope:

- are all ascending and descending strokes straight and parallel?

Size:

- are all the letters the same size?

Spacing:

- are the spaces between words the right size?

Sitting on the line:

- are the body of the letters touching the line?

Check finished writing

What did I do well?
What do I need to improve?
Refer to Handwriting self-evaluation checklist (**A2**)

OT4 Relaxation techniques for the writing hand

Students who experience difficulties when handwriting often require strategies they can frequently use in the classroom to alleviate tension and pain in the writing hand.

The following suggestions may be helpful:

- **Position hands** under thighs, flat on chair seat, palms down, rock discretely from side to side, straighten elbows, push down through hands to lift bottom off chair.

- **Place palms together and interlock fingers**, turn fingers towards body and push away with elbows straight.

- **Arms down by sides**, make a tight fist in both hands and then straighten and spread fingers.

- **Place palms of hands together** in 'prayer position' with fingers stretched then lower forearms onto table, keeping fingers pointing upwards and wrists extended.

- **Shake arms and hands** down by sides.

Occupational Therapy Approaches for Secondary Special Needs © Whurr Publishers Ltd 2002

Students who experience difficulties with fine motor dexterity and strength may benefit from regular opportunities to practise and improve fine motor skills. Collect a variety of items to make your own 'hand gym' box. For example:

- **hand grips** to squeeze in a variety of strengths (available from sports shops);
- **'theraband'** to stretch or pull against resistance;
- **stress balls** to squeeze;
- **chinese balls** to rotate within the hand;
- **therapeutic putty**/clay to roll, pinch, stretch;
- **paper clips** to make chain or place around a square of strong card;
- **travel games** with very small pegs;
- **origami** for folding and pressing;
- **bubble wrap** to pop by opposing thumb and fingers;
- **velcro strips** to pull apart and squeeze together again using pincer grip;
- **paper to tear** into strips placing it between the thumb and finger;
- **hand-held stapler** to punch and make a picture;
- **tug-of-war game** with partner:
    - make a circle with thumb and index finger, interlock with partner and pull
    - grasp cardboard tube and pull
- **hot beads and templates** to make mats, bookmarks, patterns, etc.;
- **shuffling and turning cards** when playing card games;
- **string or wool for 'cat's cradle'** using the whole hand and finger isolation;
- **scrunching paper to make balls** and flicking with thumb and each finger in turn;
- **squeezy bottles** to chase a table tennis ball around a bowl of water;
- **coin/brass rubbings**;
- **thick rubber bands** to stretch using mid-position of thumb and fingers on both hands;
- **jacks**.

It is important that students keep a record of their chosen activities and score the number of attempts to complete the challenge. They can then try to beat their own score on subsequent days.

OT6 Upper body strengthening

Upper body strength and shoulder girdle stability are essential for fluency and precision of fine motor control. Students may benefit from regular opportunities to strengthen their upper limbs. It is important that students keep a record of their chosen activities and score the number of successful attempts they have achieved.

A selection of the following suggestions may be helpful.

- **Press-ups** against the wall.

- **Modified floor push-ups**, leaving knees on the ground.

- **Modified crab walk/crab football.**

- **Squat jumps.**

- **Chair dips**:
  - (i) kneel between two chairs, one hand on each chair – push up with hands to raise body onto toes;
  - (ii) stand between two chairs placed back to back. Place one hand on the back of each chair and push up to lift body and swing legs or pull up knees and hold position to count of 10;
  - (iii) sit on chair with both hands either side of seat and slowly lower body forward to ground bending elbows. Reverse procedure to get back onto chair.

- **Mirroring games in pairs**:
  - (i) isolating index finger – Students hold opposite ends of pencil with index finger. One student moves stick whilst partner mirrors/follows the movement;
  - (ii) repeat, increasing number of fingers holding sticks;
  - (iii) repeat using other objects, e.g. ball.

- **Games in high kneeling**:
  - (i) tug-of-war;
  - (ii) tray pushing with partner – kneel opposite partner with hands flat against tray held at shoulder level. Keeping elbows straight and hands on tray, push partner;
  - (iii) ball games – throw/bounce ball above head to partner/wall.

- **Arm wrestling**:
  - (i) at table;
  - (ii) lying on tummy or floor;
  - (iii) sitting back to back, interlink arms and push each other sideways *or* push other person over line.

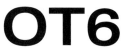

● **Shoulder resistance exercises in standing with partner**:

(i) face partner with arms out straight. One partner has both hands facing up, the other with both hands facing down. Interlink by gripping forearms. Push in direction of palms.

(ii) as above with arms facing inwards/outwards.

OT7 Self-organization

Students who experience difficulty organizing themselves throughout the day may benefit from utilizing a variety of strategies. It is essential to discuss the options with both student and parents to ensure the strategies become automatic and useful for the student. They may initially need considerable adult support, but this support/guidance can be gradually reduced as the student's independence increases.

Preparation for the school day

Using two-week timetables:

- **Use different colours to code Week 1 and Week 2,** on timetable and on a year planner at home.

Reading timetable and remembering items:

- **transfer information,** regarding e.g. sports kit, library book, musical instruments onto a weekly planner;
- **use pictures/symbols** to remind student to take specific items to school, e.g. sports kit, library book, musical instruments;
- **use a colour coding system** to identify all information relevant to a subject e.g. maths = red, English = blue. Book covers are available in different colours and will also help to protect books;
- **use checklists or post-its** on bedroom wall;
- **duplicate timetables,** e.g. home/school/locker door.

Packing school bag:

Students with poor self-organization often carry everything with them to ease their anxiety;

- **encourage student to empty bag at end of each day.** Set up an organized storage system at home, e.g. filing trays, drawer/box file, colour coded to correspond with 'colour' of subjects; have storage space for large pieces of equipment, e.g. kit, musical instruments;
- **encourage student to pack bag the night before** to reduce stress and anxiety in the morning;
- **use a checklist** and cross-check with timetable/planner;
- **purchase a school bag** suitable for student's requirements. Consider size, type, style, number and accessibility of pockets (enough to assist with organization but remember, too many cause confusion).

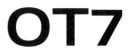

Organization within the school day

- **Self and belongings** – consider provision of a designated place (box in Learning Support, locker) for student to leave specific equipment, e.g. musical instrument, laptop, PE kit, books.

- **Lockers or a designated place** will be useful for students who prefer to carry everything everywhere. Carrying heavy bags will place excessive strain on the spine/joints of students who are already at risk, due to physical disabilities or co-ordination difficulties.

- **When working on loose sheets of paper** encourage student to write name, subject, date and number on top of each page.

- **Encourage student to file sheets at end of each lesson** by using:

  (a) coloured plastic pocket files;

  (b) exercise books covered in coloured plastic book covers;

  (c) A4 ring file with dividers coloured for each subject;

  (d) triangular cardboard pocket inserted into back of exercise book to slot work in and keep in order.

- **Ensure workplace is uncluttered.** Return equipment to correct place after use.

- **Lunch breaks** – raise staff awareness of need to support student with management of money, tray, lunch box.

Remembering important information

- **Use rough book/small pocket-sized notebook** to jot down important things to remember.

- **Make lists of things to do** and cross things off when they are done.

- **Keep post-it notes in bag/working file** to write notes to yourself. Decide on a consistent place to stick/write messages.

- **Leave clear space on timetables** for adding reminders.

- **Use transparent pencil cases** for ease of visual checking.

- **Simple check lists in 'link book'** to remind student of items they regularly need to take home e.g. blazer, laptop, PE kit, musical instrument.

Following the instructions of a task

- **Encourage student to read directions aloud** twice to ensure student has understood them.

- **Highlight directions** with a marker.

- **Check off each step as it is completed.**

Homework

- **Use a wall calendar** to record important dates or events.
- **Ensure regular homework and after-school activities** are noted on weekly timetable.
- **Use a 'plan' book** to keep track of daily/weekly/ monthly homework assignments.
- **Use a homework diary**/folder/box file.
- **Dividers could be used in a ring binder/folder** to identify days of the week and homework can be filed under the day it is due in.
- **Colour code homework** for filing according to subject.
- **Ensure student has understood and correctly recorded homework** set. If necessary provide adult/peer support so that student remembers homework.
- **Student may benefit from attending homework clubs.**

Occupational Therapy Approaches for Secondary Special Needs © Whurr Publishers Ltd 2002

Appendices

A1 Alternative methods of recording

A2 Handwriting self-evaluation checklist

A3 Information communication technology checklist and resources

A4 Teachers' checklist for visual signs

A5 Student work schedule

A6 Individual student profile

A1 Alternative methods of recording

There are many reasons why students may have difficulty recording their work, as already noted throughout this book. Students should be encouraged to experiment with some of the following strategies in order to find the most effective method/methods.

- Trial of a variety of writing tools and grips – see Occupational Therapy sheet (**OT1**) and Equipment resources (**ER**).
- Discuss with the student whether cursive or printed script is preferable.

- Experiment with different line widths of paper.
- Provide lined/squared/music staved paper/graph paper where appropriate.
- Consider allowing the student to double space their work.
- Negotiate with the student the amount of written work which is acceptable.

- Use part-prepared worksheets.
- Provide photocopied sheets.
- Encourage one line answers.
- Use tick boxes.
- Use multiple-choice questions and answers.

- Use an adult to scribe for student.
- Appoint scribe for group work to record notes for all members.
- Consider buddy working.

- Explore appropriate information communication technology, e.g. dictaphone, laptop/word processor, spell checker, calculator, etc.
- Refer to information communication technology checklist and resources (**A3**) and Equipment resources (**ER**).

Occupational Therapy Approaches for Secondary Special Needs © Whurr Publishers Ltd 2002

Observed benefits of information communication technology

- ITC enables student to keep up with peers.
- It ensures good, clear presentation of work.
- It enables student and teacher to read back what has been written.
- It increases self-confidence and self-esteem.

Always

- provide positive feedback;
- break down task into small attainable targets;
- allow extra time.

A2　Handwriting self-evaluation checklist

Name..　Class ....　Date...............

I sit correctly				YES ☐	NO ☐	
My tool hold is correct				YES ☐	NO ☐	
My non-writing hand is placed on the paper correctly				YES ☐	NO ☐	
I need to use a tool grip				YES ☐	NO ☐	

#		ALL	MOST	SOME/YES	NONE/NO
1	My letters are formed correctly	ALL ☐	MOST ☐	SOME ☐	NONE ☐
2	My tall letters are the correct height	ALL ☐	MOST ☐	SOME ☐	NONE ☐
3	My letters with tails are the correct length	ALL ☐	MOST ☐	SOME ☐	NONE ☐
4	My middle sized letters are the same size	ALL ☐	MOST ☐	SOME ☐	NONE ☐
5	My oval letters are closed	ALL ☐	MOST ☐	SOME ☐	NONE ☐
6	The straight lines of my letters are straight	ALL ☐	MOST ☐	SOME ☐	NONE ☐
7	The slant of my letters is regular (parallel)	ALL ☐	MOST ☐	SOME ☐	NONE ☐
8	My letters sit on the lines correctly	ALL ☐	MOST ☐	SOME ☐	NONE ☐
9	The spacing between my letters is even			YES ☐	NO ☐
10	The spacing between my words is even			YES ☐	NO ☐
11	My capital letters are formed correctly	ALL ☐	MOST ☐	SOME ☐	NONE ☐
12	I use my capital letters correctly			YES ☐	NO ☐
13	I use full stops correctly			YES ☐	NO ☐
14	I join letters correctly	ALL ☐	MOST ☐	SOME ☐	NONE ☐
15	My horizontal joins are correct	ALL ☐	MOST ☐	SOME ☐	NONE ☐
16	My diagonal joins are correct	ALL ☐	MOST ☐	SOME ☐	NONE ☐
17	My numbers are formed correctly	ALL ☐	MOST ☐	SOME ☐	NONE ☐

I need to work on:

1 ....

2 ....

3 ....

Taken from Taylor J (2001) Handwriting: A Teacher's Guide. London: David Fulton Publishers. Used with permission

Checklist: Seating, positioning and keyboarding skills

Name: .... Date of birth: .... Tutor group: ....

Completed by: .... Date: ....

	Yes	No
Chair Is it the right height and size? Are the student's feet on the floor or appropriately supported? Is the chair pulled up to the table?		
Table/trolley Is it the right height and size? Is there support for the forearm? Is there room for the student to work around the keyboard?		
The room Is there easy access to plugs? Is there good natural light without reflection? Will other students be distracted? Is there easy access to printer, etc.?		
The laptop Is the position/angle/height correct? Is the screen definition clear? Are there appropriate arrangements for saving, printing, recharging batteries, etc. Is the student organized enough to open/close files, print out work and save it?		
The full-size computer Is the screen at eye level? Is the screen far enough away? Is the screen in front of the student? Is the keyboard easily accessible?		

(continued)

Checklist (continued)

	Yes	No

Keyboarding skills

Does the student have good hand skills/finger awareness?

Is the student using both hands?

Is the student consistent about fingers used?

Does the student need keyboard prompts – dividing strips, lower case stickers or colour coding?

Does the keyboard response time need adjusting?

Is the student motivated to learn keyboard skills?

Is the student following a keyboarding programme?

Is there a keyboarding target in the student's individual education plan?

Other issues

Does everyone understand why the student is using the computer?

Has the student got a contract detailing when the computer is to be used?

Does the student need additional equipment, e.g. wrist support, book rest, tracker ball, etc.?

Have safety and storage issues been addressed?

Are arrangements for monitoring and assessment included in the student's individual education plan?

Who is responsible for the equipment and the supervision of its use?

How are staff kept informed and up to date?

How are the student's changing needs addressed?

Lisa Johnson ICT Inspector
Jill Jenkinson, Senior Occupational Therapist

ICT resources

It is essential that a multidisciplinary approach is adopted when students are assessed for any ICT equipment. Seek advice from your LEA ICT advisor, occupational therapist and other personnel involved.

Suggested equipment

- **Rise and fall computer tables** – can improve a student's working posture; suppliers include Varitech, Astor-Bannerman, Semerc, Inclusive Technology, GLS Dudley.

- **Wrist rest/support** – can help to reduce user fatigue; suppliers include REM, Semerc, GLS Dudley, Inclusive Technology, commercial computer stores, Posturite.

- **Key guards** – fit onto the keyboard and help students to press one key at a time; suppliers include REM, Semerc, Inclusive Technology

- **Screen filters** – can help to reduce glare; suppliers include commercial computer stores, GLS Dudley, Consortium.

- **Copyholders** – can help students copy information; suppliers include commercial computer stores, GLS Dudley, Consortium.

- **Keyboard letter stickers** – are available in a variety of letter styles and contrasts; suppliers include Inclusive Technology, REM, Semerc.

- A range of **alternative access devices** is available such as switches, mouse, joysticks, big key keyboards; suppliers include REM, Inclusive Technology, Semerc, Posturite.

Suggested software

A variety of **keyboard awareness software** is available, such as:

- Touch Type available from Semerc, Inclusive Technology;
- Ultrakey, Type to Learn, Iota Touch Type, Kaz, Mavis Beacon Teaches Typing 9; all available from REM;
- Five Finger Typist available from Inclusive Technology.

A variety of software/programs with **word lists/word banks** is available, such as:

- Clicker – available from REM, Semerc;
- Inclusive Writer – available from REM, Inclusive Technology;
- Wordbar – available from REM

A variety of software/programs with **prediction utilities**, which display wordlists based on a combination of initial letters, is available, such as:

- Predict IT – available from REM, Semerc;
- Penfriend – available from REM, Semerc, Inclusive Technology.

Adaptations/strategies to try

- **Double spacing** of text may be achieved by setting this as a default.

- **Dampening of keys** – autorepeat facility can be adjusted to stop letters repeating themselves across the screen if key is depressed for too long. Or go to control panel and select keyboard then change rate of repeat keys to slow.

- **Text to speech facility** can be set to read back what has been written. Consider use of an ear piece.

- If student has difficulty reading information presented in different font styles use consistent styles by setting up in control panel and user in PC.

- If student prefers to use a mouse instead of a keyboard an on screen keyboard may be useful.

Useful contacts

ACE (Aiding Communication in Education)
Centre Advisory Trust
92 Windmill Road
Headington
Oxford OX3 7DR
Tel: 01865 759800
Email: info@ace-centre.org.uk
www.ace-centre.org.uk – a variety of
information sites are available on the
website.

ACE Centre Advisory Trust – North
1 Broadbent Road
Watersheddings
Oldham
OL1 4HU
Tel: 0161 6271385
Email: ace-north@ace-north.org
www.ace-centre.org.uk

The ACE Centres provide a focus for the use of technology for the communication and educational needs of young people with physical impairments and communication difficulties. A wide variety of services is available including assessment, information and specialist training.

CALL Centre
University of Edinburgh Patterson's Land
Hollyrood
Edinburgh
EH8 8AQ
Tel: 0131 6516236
Email: call.centre@ed.ac.uk
www.callcentrescotland.org.uk

Don Johnson Special Needs Ltd
18/19 Clarendon Court
Winwick Quay
Warrington WA2 8QP
www.donjohnson.com – a variety of
information sites are available on the
website.
A catalogue is also available

Keytools Ltd
PO Box 700
Southampton SO17 1LQ
Tel: 023 8058 431114
Email: info@keytools.com
www.keytools.com – a variety of
information sites are available.

Becta
Milburn Hill Road
Science Park
Coventry
CV4 7JJ
www.becta.org.uk – provides
information, advice and dialogue
relating to ICT and education for
schools.

Teachers' checklist for visual signs

A4

Child's name: ....

Form/Teacher reference: ....

1   **Please circle the special areas (if any) of difficulty this child has with reading:**

Vocabulary   Word recognition   Oral reading   Silent reading   Rate
Interpretation   Attention   Comprehension

2   **Four classifications of frequency of performance traits are given:**

A   Meaning very often observed (many times/day)
B   Meaning regularly observed (daily)
C   Meaning sometimes observed
D   Meaning seldom observed

3   **Please ring the letter you best consider indicates the child's performance.**

Does the child show any of the following?

a	Skipping or rereading lines or words	A	B	C	D
b	Reads too slowly	A	B	C	D
c	Uses finger or marker as pointer when reading	A	B	C	D
d	Lacks ability to remember what he has read	A	B	C	D
e	Shows fatigue or listlessness when reading	A	B	C	D
f	Complains of print 'running together' or 'jumping'	A	B	C	D
g	Gets too close to reading and writing tasks	A	B	C	D
h	Loss of attention to task at hand	A	B	C	D
i	Distracted by other activities	A	B	C	D
j	Assumes an improper or awkward sitting position	A	B	C	D
k	Writes crookedly, poor spaced letters, cannot stay on ruled lines, excessive pressure used	A	B	C	D
l	Orientates drawings poorly on paper	A	B	C	D
m	Is seen to blink frequently	A	B	C	D
n	Rubs eyes excessively	A	B	C	D

General observations:

o	Clumsiness and difficulty manipulating own body and other objects in space available, including problems with ball control	A	B	C	D
p	Awareness of things around him in the classroom to point where he turns to look at stimulus	A	B	C	D
q	Is this child able to maintain his involvement with your instruction?	A	B	C	D

Scoring

Any scores of 'A', more than two scores of 'B' and more than three or four scores of 'C' suggest that prompt referral to an optometrist specializing in children's eye care is indicated. A copy of this checklist would also be helpful to the optometrist.

Taken from Holland K (1995) Visual Skills for Learning in Topic, Spring, No 13. NFER-NELSON. Used with permission.

Students with autistic spectrum disorder need visual ways of understanding what they have to do. This work schedule incorporates the TEACCH principle to enable teachers to provide students with clear guidelines.

It was developed for use with Asperger students in mainstream schools who were not completing tasks set by staff, both in lessons and for homework.

It has a general application for children with other medical conditions presenting the same difficulties.

A blank proforma of the work schedule has been provided to enable staff to use this technique with students.

Reference

Schopler E, Mesibov GB, Hearsey K (1995) Structured teaching in the TEACCH system, in Schopler E, Mesibov GB (eds) *Learning and Cognition in Autism*. New York: Plenum Press.

A5 Student work schedule

Example of a work schedule

Name: ....   Date of Birth: ....   Tutor Group: ....

Subject: ....   Task/Topic: ....   Teacher: ....

What work?	How much work?	How will I know it is finished?	What next?
Details of content, e.g. written exercise? Essay? Questions to be answered? Independent reading? etc.	Quantity of work, amount of writing, number of questions, time allowed, etc.	Details of how it will be assessed, mark allocation, how will teacher monitor what I have done?	If work completed satisfactorily what will next 'work' be? If unsatisfactory what will happen?
Piece of creative writing titled ' . . .'	1 side of A4 lined paper	- amount of writing - satisfactory standard - on the subject	Break time
OR			
Worksheet on Queen Victoria Twentieth Century	Answer all the questions.	- all answered answers - at least 15/20 correct	Start project on the - complete sentences for
OR			
Reading book ' . . .' (homework)	spend half an hour this evening reading	- check times (get witness?) - be ready to say what you read about	own choice

Alison Reevey, Fosseway School, Midsomer Norton, Bath and North East Somerset.

236

A5

Work schedule

Name: ....   Date of Birth: ....   Tutor Group: ....

Subject: ....   Task/Topic: ....   Teacher: ....

What work?	How much work?	How will I know it is finished?	What next?

A6 Individual student profile

The following profile has been developed to enable special educational needs co-ordinators or teachers to identify the key problem areas affecting a particular student's performance within the classroom or wider school environment. A blank proforma of the individual student profile has been provided for staff to complete.

Observed behaviours can be recorded in the first column and appropriate practical strategies selected from the relevant medical condition/curriculum tables listed in the second column. The individual responsible for implementation can be noted in the third column and the place and/or time for that implementation written in the fourth column. A final column has been included to evaluate the outcome.

Example of an individual student profile sheet

Individual student profile

Name: .... Date of Birth: .... Tutor Group: ....

Medical condition: .... Subject: ....

Completed by: .... Date: ....

Observed Behaviour	Practical Strategies	Who will implement?	When?	Outcome
Reduced stamina for extended periods of writing	• Pre-prepared worksheets	• Adult support	• Prior to lesson	• More focused in class and able to keep up with peers
Carrying dangerous equipment e.g. knives	Stage 1 • Undertake risk assessment Stage 2 • Implement risk assessment recommendations, e.g. provide own set of tools	• Health and safety rep./ teacher • Teacher/adult support	• As soon as possible • In class during practical lesson	• Form completed – move to Stage 2 • Highlighted student still dangerous with knife so repeat risk assessment
Difficulty finding place on board	• Use different coloured pens • Keep board as uncluttered as possible • Provide desk top copy of information	• Teacher • Teacher • Teacher/adult support	• During lesson • During lesson • Prior to lesson	• Too time-consuming for teacher – broke up 'flow' of lesson • Student able to follow lesson more easily • Student able to find place and keep up with peers

A6

Example of an individual student profile sheet

Name: ....

Date of Birth: ....

Tutor Group: ....

Medical condition: ....

Subject: ....

Completed by: ....

Date: ....

Observed Behaviour	Practical Strategies	Who will implement?	When?	Outcome

240

Equipment resources

This section lists a variety of sources for equipment mentioned throughout the book. In addition to the suppliers' names most areas now have a local shop selling equipment for the disabled where it is possible to try equipment before purchasing. There is also a network of Independent Living Centres throughout the country (listed in Yellow Pages®). These often have an occupational therapist on the staff who can advise on suitable equipment. For addresses and phone numbers for the suppliers listed below refer to the end of this chapter.

Equipment	Suppliers
Angled work surfaces Write-angle – Desktop writing aid Writestart desktop Posturite board, clear perspex writing slope Book rests Reference holder Copy holder Posture pack (writing slope and seat wedge)	Philip and Tacey LDA Posturite UK Ltd Kitchen Stores GLS Educational Supplies, Computer Accessory Shops Back In Action, Children's Seating Centre
Calculators Desktop calculators	HOPE, Consortium, GLS Educational Supplies
Compasses Beam compass (Helix) easy to use Circle master – compass and protractor in one Safe drawing compass	Philip and Tacey, GLS Educational Supplies

Computer-related equipment
Typing/keyboard skills software:
    Touch Type
    Ultrakey
    Type to Learn
    Iota Touch Type
    Five Finger Typist
    Mavis Beacon Teaches Typing 9
    Clicker 4
    Predict IT
    Penfriend
    Inclusive Writer
    Word Bar
    Easy Type 2 Typing Programme
    Keyguard
    Wrist Supports
	
	Semerc
	REM
	REM
	REM
	Inclusive Technology
	REM
	REM
	REM, Semerc
	REM, Semerc
	REM, Semerc
	REM
	Egon Publishers
	REM, Semerc
	REM, Semerc, GLS Educational Supplies

Equipment	Suppliers
Dictionaries ACE	LDA
Kitchen equipment *Tap turners* – there are two main types of tap tuners to fit either capstan/crosshead or crystal taps.	Keep Able, Nottingham Rehabilitation
Bread buttering boards – help stabilize bread for one-handed spreading. A variety is available.	Nottingham Rehabilitation, Homecraft Ability One
Tin openers, electric or manual, are available and can be free-standing or wall-mounted.	Nottingham Rehabilitation, Keep Able, Homecraft Ability One, GLS Educational Supplies
Jar openers – there is a range of products designed to make opening jars easier.	Keep Able, Homecraft Ability One, Nottingham Rehabilitation
Belly clamps – a devise which stabilizes an object using body weight	Homecraft Ability One
Kitchen knives: Knives that provide an upright handle to retain the natural position of the hand and wrist so that cutting can be whole arm action. Knives with a rocking action for ease of use.	Nottingham Rehabilitation Nottingham Rehabilitation, Homecraft Ability One, Keep Able
Peelers and graters that stabilize food and/or utensil for one-handed cutting or chopping.	Nottingham Rehabilitation, Homecraft Ability One, Keep Able
Cooking baskets – hold vegetables whilst cooking for easy removal and straining.	Nottingham Rehabilitation, Homecraft Ability One,
Trays – for carrying with one hand.	Homecraft Ability One
Kettle tippers – provide a tilting platform, which enable pouring from kettle or teapot without lifting.	Keep Able, Nottingham Rehabilitation
Turners – for small items, e.g. cooker knobs, cupboard handles.	Homecraft Ability One, Nottingham Rehabilitation
Pan handle holder – attaches to the side of the cooker and holds handle/pan in place whilst stirring.	Homecraft Ability One, Nottingham Rehabilitation

Equipment	Suppliers
Paper Paper with raised lines to assist with placement, e.g. Right Line paper, Stop-Go paper, heavily lined stationery, music stave paper	GLS Educational Supplies Taskmaster Partially-Sighted Society
Pen grips Triangular, Trigo, Grippies/Stubbi, Comfort Grips	Consortium, HOPE, LDA, Taskmaster
Pencils Pencils with a triangular shaft, e.g. Berol Handhuggers, Writestart. Pencils with an integral grip, e.g. Pilot	Consortium, HOPE, Commercial Stationers
Pens Pens with integral grips and different diameters of shaft, e.g. Berol Handhugger, Pilot Dr Grip.	Commercial Stationers, GLS Educational Supplies
Protractors Anglemaster – combined with set square, ruler. Angle Measure Circle – compass and protractor in one	Philip and Tacey, GLS Educational Supplies
Rulers Non-slip 'Super' ruler Ridgeback ruler with raised handle Decorators ruler Non-slip safety rule for design & technology	London Graphic Centre Commercial Stationers Specialist Decorators Stores GLS Educational Supplies
Scanning Line tracker	Taskmaster
Scissors Self-opening scissors Easy grip scissors Roll-cut Rotary cutter Compass cutter – cuts circles from 10 mm to 150 mm diameter	Peta, Taskmaster, GLS Educational Supplies Consortium, HOPE, GLS Educational Supplies Taskmaster Philip and Tacey, GLS Educational Supplies GLS Educational Supplies
Spell checkers Pocket Collins Dictionary Desktop Thesaurus Plus	REM

Equipment	Suppliers
Stencils	
Shapes	GLS Educational Supplies
Letters	
Electronic stencils for electronic equipment	
Flowchart – computer technology template	
Ellipse – design & technology equipment	
Letter stencils in variety of styles	Consortium
Graphic template	Consortium
Geography stencils	Consortium
Chemistry stencils	Consortium
Tables and chairs	
Rise and fall table (with tilting surface)	Panilet, Atkinson Vari-tech, Astor-Bannerman Ltd
Vela Krumme (typing chair)	Alton Aids Mobility
Classmate (typing chair)	Rainbow Rehabilitation
Perching/household stool, angled seat, variable height	Nottingham Rehabilitation
Stick stools – either canvas or travel stick style.	Homecraft Ability One, Outdoor/Camping Shops
Science stools with footrests and/or backrests.	Consortium, GLS Educational Supplies,
Tripp Trapp chair.	Nottingham Rehabilitation, Back In Action
Miscellaneous	
Trolley – walker trolleys enable safe transfer of food or heavy items from one room to another	Keep Able, Homecraft Ability One, Nottingham Rehabilitation
Needle threaders – for sewing machines or needles, alternatively a cork can be used to hold the needle.	Homecraft Ability One, Nottingham Rehab
Magnifiers – can be free-standing or around the neck.	Craft Suppliers, GLS Educational Supplies
G-Clamps to stabilize equipment on a bench or table.	DIY Stores, GLS Educational Supplies
Dycem – non-slip materials, available in rolls or mats.	Nottingham Rehabilitation, Homecraft Ability One
Rubberzote – soft padding to enlarge handles.	Nottingham Rehabilitation, Homecraft Ability One
Lego Technic Cards	Toy Shops, Educational Supplies Catalogues

Equipment	Suppliers
Miscellaneous (contined)	
Wedge cushion:	
Gymnic Movin'Sit Senior Cushion.	Epsan Waterfly (UK) Ltd
Posture Pack Seating Wedge.	Back In Action
Theraband	Physiomed, Nottingham Rehabilitation
Therapeutic Putty	Physiomed, Nottingham Rehabilitation
Lycra fabric and equipment	JABADAO

Suppliers' addresses

All of these companies supply goods throughout the UK. Some have regional representatives.

Alton Aids Mobility
Unit 31
Team Valley Business Centre
Earls Way
Team Valley Trading Estate
Gateshead
Tyne and Wear
NE11 0RQ
Tel: 0191 4915840
Email: alton.aids@virgin.net
www.altonaids.co.uk

Ann Arbor Publishers
PO Box 1
Belford
Northumberland
NE70 7JX
Tel: 01668 214460
Email: enquiries@annarbor.co.uk

Anything Left Handed Ltd
Head office/ Mail order
18 Avenue Road
Belmont
Surrey
SM2 6JD
Tel: 0208 770 3722
Email:
enquiries@anythingleft-
handed.co.uk
www.anythingleft-handed.co.uk

ASCO Educational Supplies Ltd
19 Lochwood Way
Leeds
LS11 5TH
Tel: 0113 2707070
Email: tom@binder.tele2.co.uk

Astor-Bannerman Ltd
Unit 11F
Coln Park
Andoversford
Cheltenham
GL54 4LB
Tel: 01242 820820
www.astor-bannerman.co.uk

Atkinson Vari–Tech Ltd
Unit 4
Sett End Road
Shadsworth
Blackburn
Lancashire
BB1 2PT
Tel: 01254 678777
Email:
atkinson.varitech@btinternet.com
www.vari-tech.co.uk

Back in Action
11 Whitcomb Street
London
WC2H 7HA
Tel: 0207 9308308
Email: info@backinaction.co.uk
www.backinaction.co.uk

Bath Institute of Medical Engineering
The Wolfson Centre
Royal United Hospital
Combe Park
Bath
BA1 3NG
Tel: 01225 824103
Email: mailto:bime@bath.ac.uk
www.bath.ac.uk.\centres\bime

Consortium
Consortium South West
PO Box 1170
Trowbridge
BA14 8XX
Tel: 01225 771320
Email: orders@theconsortium.co.uk
www.theconsortium.co.uk

Egon Publications
Royston Road
Baldock
Hertfordshire
SG7 6NW
Tel: 01462 894498
Email: information@egon.co.uk
www.egon.co.uk

Epsan Waterfly (UK) Ltd
Anglo House
Worcester Road
Stourport on Severn
DY13 9AW
Tel: 01299 829213
Email: salesuk@epsanwaterfly.com

Galt Educational and Pre-school
Hyde Buildings
Ashton Road
Hyde
Cheshire
SK14 4SH
Tel: 0161 8825300
Email: enquiries@galt-educational.co.uk
www.hope-education.co.uk

GLS Educational Supplies Ltd
1 Mollison Avenue
Enfield
EN3 7XQ
Tel: 0208 8058333
Email: sales@glsed.co.uk
www.glsed.co.uk

Hope Education
Hyde Buildings
Ashton Road
Hyde
Cheshire
SK14 4SH
Tel: 08702 433400
Email: enquiries@hope-educational.co.uk
www.hope-education.co.uk

Inclusive Technology Ltd
Gatehead Business Park
Delph
Oldham
OL3 5BX
Tel: 01457 819790
Email: inclusive@inclusive.co.uk
www.inclusive.co.uk

JABADAO
Branch House
18 Branch Road
Armley
Leeds
West Yorkshire
LS12 3AQ
Tel: 0113 2310650
Email: info@jabadao.org
www.jabadao.org

Keep Able Ltd
11-17 Kingston Road
Staines
Middlesex
TW18 4QX
Tel: 01784 440044
Email: sales@keepable.co.uk
www.keepable.co.uk

LDA (Learning Development Aids)
Duke Street
Wisbech
Cambridgeshire
PE13 2AE
Tel: 01945 463441
Email: ldaorders@compuserve.com
www.ldalearning.com

London Graphic Centre
16-18 Shelton Street
Covent Garden
London
WC2H 9JL
Tel: 020 7759 4500
Email:
mailorder@londongraphics.co.uk
www.londongraphics.co.uk

MSL Ltd. (Multi Sensory Learning)
Highgate House
Creaton
Northamptonshire
NN6 8NN
Tel: 01604 505000
Email: info@msl-online.net
www.msl-online.net

NFER-NELSON
Darville House
2 Oxford Road East
Windsor
Berkshire
SL4 1 DF
Tel: 01753 858961
Email: edu&hsc@nfer-nelson.co.uk
www.information@nfer-nelson.co.uk

Nottingham Rehab Supplies
Norvara House
Excelsior Road
Ashby de la Zouch
Leicestershire
LE65 1NG
Tel: 0845 120 4522
Email: info@nrs-uk.co.uk
www.information@nrs-uk.co.uk

Panilet
Unit 17
Dragoncourt
Crofts End Road
St George
Bristol
BS5 7XX
Tel: 0117 9511858

Partially Sighted Society
PO Box 322
Doncaster
South Yorkshire
DN1 2XA
Tel: 01302 323132
Email: info@partsight.org.uk

Peta (UK) Ltd
Marks Hall
Margaret Roding
Dunmow
CM6 1QT
Tel: 01245 231118
Email: sales@peta-uk.com
www.peta-uk.com

Philip and Tacey
North Way
Andover
Hants
SP10 5BA
Tel: 01264 332171
Email: sales@philipandtacey.co.uk
www.philipandtacey.co.uk

Physio Med Services Ltd
Unit 7-11
Glossopbrook Buisiness Park
Surrey Street
Glossop
Derbyshire
SK13 7AJ
Tel: 01457 860444
Email: sales@physio-med.com
www.physio-med.com

Posturite (UK) Ltd
10 Diplocks Way
Hailsham
East Sussex
BN27 3JF
Tel: 01323 847777
Email: support@posturite.co.uk
www.posturite.co.uk

Promedics Ltd (North Coast Medical)
Moorgate Street
Blackburn
BB2 4PB
Tel: 01254 619000
Email: enquiries@promedics.co.uk
www.promedics.co.uk

Rainbow Rehabilitation
Scandic Rehab
The Coach House
134 Purewell
Christchurch
Dorset
BH23 1EU
Tel: 01202 481818
www.rainbow-rehab.co.uk

REM (Rickitt Educational Media Ltd)
Great Western House
Langport
Somerset
TA10 9YU
Tel: 01458 254700
Email: sales@r-e-m.co.uk
www.r-e-m.co.uk

SEMERC
Granada Learning – SEMERC
Granada Television
Quay Street
Manchester
M60 9EA
Tel: 0161 8272887
Email: info@granada-learning.com
www. granada-learning.com

Smart Kids (UK) Ltd
169B Main Street
New Greenham Park
Thatcham
Berks
RG19 6HN
Tel: 01635 44037
Email: sales@smartkids.co.uk
www.smartkidscatalog.com

Homecraft Ability One Ltd
Shelly Close
Lowmoor Road Industrial Estate
Kirkby-in-Ashfield
Nottinghamshire
NG17 7ET
Tel: 01623 720005

Tarquin Publication
Stradbroke
Diss
Norfolk
IP21 5JP
Tel: 01379 384218
Email: enquiries@tarquin-
books.demon.co.uk
www.tarquin-books.demon.co.uk

Taskmaster Ltd
Morris Road
Leicester
LE2 6BR
Tel: 0116 2704286
Email: info@taskmasteronline.co.uk
www.taskmasteronline.co.uk

The Happy Puzzle Company
PO Box 24041
London
NW4 2ZN
Tel: 0208 2027770
Email: info@happypuzzle.co.uk
www.happypuzzle.co.uk

Winslow
Goyt Side Road
Chesterfield
Derbyshire
S40 2PH
Tel: 0848 921 1777
Email: sales@winslow-cat.com

Useful addresses

ACE Centre Advisory Trust
92 Windmill Road
Headington
Oxford
OX3 7DR
Tel: 01865 759800
Email: info@ace-centre.org.uk
www.ace-centre.org.uk

(Provides a focus for the use of technology with the communication and educational needs of young people with physical impairments and communication difficulties.)

ACE Centre North
1 Broadbent Road
Watersheddings
Oldham
OL1 4HU
Tel: 0161 627 1358
Email: enquiries@ace-north.org.uk
www.ace-centre.org.uk

Association of Paediatric Chartered Physiotherapist
See: The Chartered Society of Physiotherapists

Bath Institute of Medical Engineering (BIME)
The Wolfson Centre
Royal United Hospital
Combe Park
Bath
BA1 3NG
Tel: 01225824103
Email: bime@bath.ac.uk
www.bath.ac.uk\centres\bime

(Design and technology charity interested in developing devices that have a general application.)

Becta (British Educational Communications and Technology Agency)
Millburn Hill Road
Science Park
Coventry
CV4 7JJ
Tel: 02476 41 6994
Email: becta@becta.org.uk
www.becta.org.uk

(Website provides information, advice and dialogue relating to ICT and education for schools.)

British Association of Occupational Therapists
(College of Occupational Therapists)
106-114 Borough High Street
Southwark
London
SE1 1LB
Tel: 020 7357 6480
www.cot.co.uk

British Dyslexia Association
98 London Road
Reading
RG1 5AU
Tel: 0118 966 2677 (admin)
Tel: 0118 966 8271 (helpline)
Email: admin@bda-dyslexia.demon.co.uk
info@dyslexiahelp-bda.demon.co.uk
www.bda-dyslexia.org.uk

Occupational Therapy Approaches for Secondary Special Needs © Whurr Publishers Ltd 2002

CALL (Communication Aids for Language and Learning) Centre
University of Edinburgh
Patersen's Land
Holyrood Road
Edinburgh
EH8 8AQ
Tel: 0131 651 6236
Email: call.centre@ed.ac.uk
www.callcentrescotland.org.uk

(Provides specialist expertise for children who have speech, communication and/or writing difficulties in schools across Scotland.)

The Chartered Society of Physiotherapy
14 Bedford Row
Chancery Lane
London
WC1R 4ED
Tel: 0207 306 6666
Email: csp@csphysio.org.uk
www.csp.org.uk

Contact a Family (UK Office)
209-211 City Road
London
EC1V IJN
Tel: 0207 608 8700
Helpline: 08088 083555
Email: info@cafamily.org.uk
www.cafamily.org.uk

(Provide a directory of specific conditions and rare syndromes in children with their family support networks. They also have a website and helpline.)

Handwriting Interest Group
Membership Secretary
5 River Meadow
Hemingford Abbot
Huntingdon
PE28 9AY
www.handwritinginterestgroup.org.uk

(Set up to raise standards in the teaching of handwriting in schools and to disseminate teaching ideas and methods.)

National Association of Paediatric Occupational Therapists (NAPOT)
65 Prestbury Road
Wilmslow
Cheshire
SK9 2LL
Tel: 01625 549266
Email: htidey@napot-u-net.com

Questions Publishing
27 Frederick Street
Birmingham
B1 3HH
Tel: 0121 2120919
Email: webmaster@questpub.co.uk
www.education-quest.com

(Publish a range of magazines covering literacy, maths, science, school management, ICT, thinking skills, PE, special needs.)

Royal College of Speech and Language Therapists
2 Whiteheart Yard
London
SE1 1NX
Tel: 0207 3781200
Email: postmaster@rcslt.org
www.rcslt.org

REMAP
(Registered national charity that designs and makes technical equipment for disabled people.)

National Organizer REMAP
J.J. Wright
Hazeldene
Ighiham
Sevenoaks
Kent
TN15 9AD
Tel: 08451 300456
Email: john.wright@remap.org.uk
www.remap.org.uk

National Organizer REMAP
(Northern Ireland)
Victor Cole
4 Golden View Park
Greenisland
BT38 8RS
Tel: 02890 864251
Email: victor.cole@btinternet.com

National Organizer REMAP
(Scotland)
Mr J Golder
Maulside Lodge
Beith
Ayrshire
KA15 1JJ
Tel: 01294 832566
Email: scotland@remap.org.uk

SENCO Update
Optimus Publishing
Freepost LON 13693
67-71 Goswell Road
London
EC1B 1LT
www.optimuspub.co.uk

(Monthly newsletter written specifically to
provide news, analysis and practical guidance
for SENCOs.)

Further reading

Circle of Friends

Maines B, Robinson G (1998) All for Alex. A Circle of Friends. Bristol: Lucky Duck.

Taylor G (1997) Community building in schools: developing a circle of friends. Educational and Child Psychology 14: 45-50.

Whittaker P, Barrett P, Joy H, Potter M and Thomas G (1998) Children with autism and peer group support: using Circle of Friends. British Journal of Special Education 25(2): 60-64.

Diagnostic criteria

American Psychiatric Association (1995) Diagnostic and Statistical Manual of Mental Disorders: DSMVI: International Version with ICD 10 Codes, 4th edn. Washington, DC: The American Psychiatric Association.

World Health Organization (1992,1993,1994) International Statistical Classification of Diseases and Related Health Problems, 10th revision, 3 vols. Geneva: World Health Organization.

Educational inclusion

Farrell M (2000) Educational inclusion and raising standards. British Journal of Special Education 27(1): 35-38.

Mackey S, McQueen J (1998) Exploring the association between integrated therapy and inclusive education. British Journal of Special Education 25(1): 22-27.

Mitler P (2000) Working Towards Inclusive Education. London: Fulton.

Gross motor activities

Russell JP (1988) Graded Activities for Children with Motor Difficulties. Cambridge: Cambridge University Press.

Elphinston J, Pook P (1998) The Core Workout – A Definitive Guide to Swiss Ball Training for Athletes, Coaches and Fitness Professionals. Fleet: Core Workouts, Rugby Science.

Mind mapping

Buzan T (1989) Use Your Head. London: BBC Publications.

Russell P (1984) The Brain Book. New York: Dutton.

Social stories

Gray C (1994) Comic Strip Conversations: Colorful, Illustrated Interactions with Students with Autism and Related Disorders. Jenison, MI: Jenison Public Schools.

Gray C (1997) Social Stories and Comic Strip Conversations. Arlington, TX: Future Horizons.

Gray C (1998) Social Stories and Comic Strip Conversations – Unique Methods to Improve Understanding (video). Arlington, TX: Future Horizons.

Gray C (2000) The New Social Story Book. Arlington, TX: Future Horizons.

TEACCH

Schopler E, Mesibov GB, Hearsey K (1995) Structured teaching in the TEACCH system, in Schopler E, Mesibov GB (eds) Learning and Cognition in Autism. New York: Plenum Press.

The National Curriculum

Department for Education and Employment (1999) The National Curriculum. Handbook for Secondary Teachers in England. London: Department for Education and Employment.

Writing frames

Lewis M, Wray D (1998) Writing across the Curriculum: Frames to Support Learning. Reading: University of Reading.

Wray D, Lewis M (1997) Extending Literacy: Children's Reading and Writing Non-fiction. London: Routledge.

Glossary

Amanuensis Someone who writes from dictation.

Asymmetrical Where one side of the body differs from the other.

Ataxia Movements are jerky, unsteady, walking with a wide base, imperfect balance and at times an intention tremor.

Atrophy Wasting of muscles or nerve cells.

Bilateral integration The ability to use two sides of the body together in a co-ordinated manner.

Child and adolescent mental health service (CAMHS) This is a service for children and families with emotional and behavioural problems. It is usually a multidisciplinary team offering a variety of therapies. The team may include: psychiatrist, clinical psychologist, occupational therapist, community psychiatric nurse, play therapist, social worker, psychotherapist.

Congenital Existing at or before birth.

Contracture Permanently tight muscles and joints.

Dislocation The displacement of one or more bones of a joint from the original position.

DT Design technology.

Dynamic balance The ability to maintain balance whilst moving, e.g. walking, roller-blading.

Dyspraxia Difficulty in planning and carrying out skilled, non-habitual motor acts in the correct sequence.

Dystonia Fluctuating, variable tone.

Extension The process of straightening or stretching the body or a limb.

Flexion Bending or pulling in a part of the body.

Hypertonia High muscle tone, which often results in a degree of tightness.

Hypotonia Low muscle tone, which often results in a degree of floppiness.

ICT Information communication technology.

LEA Local Education Authority/Education Library Boards (Northern Ireland).

Lordosis Forward curvature of the spine.

Motor planning The ability of the brain to conceive of, organize and carry out a sequence of unfamiliar or unskilled motor actions.

Occupational Therapy (OT) is the treatment of physical and psychiatric conditions through specific activities to help people reach their maximum level of function and independence in all aspects of daily life (World Federation of Occupational Therapists).

PE Physical education.

Proximal Nearest to the body.

Proprioception The ability to know where body parts are in space without looking/using vision. Proprioceptors are found in muscles, joints and tendons.

Remediation is intervention designed to help a person to learn certain functional skills that may have been incompletely or inaccurately learnt.

Saccadic eye movements are those made when eyes selectively jump from one place to another e.g. when moving from one fixation point on a page to another during reading.

Scoliosis A sideways curvature of the spine.

Sensory modulation When an individual over-responds, under-responds or fluctuates in response to sensory input in a manner disproportional to that input.

SENCO Special educational needs co-ordinator/Learning support services (Scotland).

Splint A support made for joints that are inflamed, to rest and maintain them in a functional position.

Static balance The ability to maintain balance whilst standing still, e.g. standing on one leg whilst putting on a shoe.

Subluxation A partial dislocation.

Symmetrical When both sides of the body are the same.

Tactile defensivity A dysfunction where tactile sensations cause excessive emotional reactions, hyperactivity or other behavioural problems. The person can feel discomfort and a desire to escape the situation when certain types of tactile stimuli are experienced.

Tone The normal tensions of the muscles at rest.

Tremor A very fine kind of jerking spasm.

Vestibular system The sensory system that responds to the position of the head in relation to gravity and accelerated or decelerated movement.

Index

art 175–86; problems with:
 auditory processing and memory
  185–6
 fine motor dexterity 177–9
 gross motor co-ordination 175–7
 organizational skills 179–80
 social interaction 186
 visual closure 184
 visual figure ground discrimination
  182–3
 visual form constancy 184
 visual memory/sequential memory 185
 visual motor integration 181
 visual spatial relationships 181–2
Asperger's syndrome 35, 46–54
 co-morbidity 46
 see also autistic spectrum disorders
ataxic cerebral palsy 55
athetoid cerebral palsy 55
attentional deficit disorder/attention
  hyperactivity disorder 35, 36–45
 behaviour 40
 diagnosis 36
 fine motor dexterity 42
 gross motor skills 41
 management approaches 40–5
 organizational skills 42
 perception 44
 presenting features 37, 40–5
 self-care 44
 social skills 45
 treatment 38
auditory perception 14
auditory processing and memory 30–31
  implications for:
 art 185–6
 design and technology 139–40
 English 104–5
 geography 166–7
 history 154
 information communication
  technology 145
 mathematics 115–16
 modern foreign languages 174
 music 192
 physical education 201
 science 126–7
autistic spectrum disorders 35, 46–54
 behaviours 50
 communication 53
 diagnosis 46
 fine motor dexterity 51
 gross motor skills 51
 management approaches 50–4
 organizational skills 52

 presenting feature 46–7, 50–4
 response to sensory input 50
 social skills 54
 treatment 47

balance 2, 10, 13
Becker muscular dystrophy 79
behaviour *see* social interaction;
   social/emotional/psychological skills
behavioural optometrist 17
bilateral integration 10
body
 awareness 2, 10, 12
 language 32

cerebral palsy 35, 55–65
 classification 55
 health 60
 management approaches 60–65
 fine motor dexterity 62
 mobility 61
 ocular motor control 64
 posture 61
 presenting features 56–7, 60–5
 prognosis 57
 self-care 63
 speech 64
 treatment 57
 visual perception 64
 weight gain 60
classroom performance 9
Codes of Practice 1
cognitive ability/skills 2, 26
communication 32
 and ADD/ADHD 43
 and autistic spectrum disorders 53
 and cerebral palsy 64
 and developmental co-ordination
  disorder 72–3
 and sequencing 14
co-morbidity 35
computer
 see information communication
  technology
conceptualization 26
confidence 11, 45
 and see self-esteem

danger, reduced sense of
 and ADD/ADHD 41, 43
 and autistic spectrum disorders 52
 and developmental co-ordination
  disorder 70

Occupational Therapy Approaches for Secondary Special Needs © Whurr Publishers Ltd 2002

Index